## Praise for *The Secret P*

"This sweetly voiced explication of the Yoga Su[...]
ity, charming and inviting the reader into the [...]
he is actually a manifestation of the Divine. I read it smiling all the way, and
learning yoga philosophy as I was doing it."
    —SYLVIA BOORSTEIN, author of *Pay Attention, for Goodness' Sake:*
    *The Buddhist Path of Kindness*

"Nischala Joy Devi has provided a dynamic new interpretation of the Yoga
Sutras, one of the most important but esoteric guidebooks to deeper Yoga
practice, that will make this wonderful ancient teaching accessible to modern
readers and useful in their daily life. She has explained the essence of Yoga in
a simple, direct, and relevant manner for all sincere students of the spiritual
path."
    —DAVID FRAWLEY (VAMADEVA SHASTRI), author of *Yoga and Ayurveda*

"Weaving together her deep knowledge of the Yoga Sutras with her many
years of teaching and studying, Nischala Devi has created a very readable and
insightful book. Her words ring with the authenticity of a committed practitioner, and the exercises she offers the reader can be truly life changing. But
I must admit, I loved her funny and inspiring stories the best! A book to be
read again and again."
    —JUDITH HANSON LASATER, PhD, PT, Yoga teacher since 1971 and
    author of six books, including *A Year of Living Your Yoga*

"Nischala Devi has given us a fresh and compelling new look into the mysteries of one of yoga's most important scriptures. Bravo! I heartily recommend
her new book to all who want to understand (and trod) the practical path of
liberation so brilliantly described by Sri Patanjali."
    —STEPHEN COPE, author of *The Wisdom of Yoga: A Seeker's Guide to*
    *Extraordinary Living*

"This book has the feel of divinely guided inspiration. A loving call to every
woman who walks the sacred journey. Nischala Joy Devi breathes new life,
enthusiasm, creativity, and insights into the endless secret powers of yoga."
    —LILIAS FOLAN, PBS host and author of *Lilias! Yoga Gets Better with Age*

"Devi boldly reinterprets the Yoga Sutras of Patanjali from a personal acknowledgment of feminine intuition. Many women will find it refreshingly accessible and uniquely relevant to their spiritual quest on the Yogic path. Nischala
brings a delightful emphasis on the celebratory Divine, inviting readers to

allow this liberating text and the visualizations she's added, to illumine our own sacred journey to the heart."

—SARAH POWERS, international Yoga and mindfulness teacher

"A wise woman's guide to a life of peace and harmony. Full of heart and with a beautiful earthy wisdom, Nischala Joy Devi has crafted a whole new and feminine dimension to these ancient writings, bringing the age-old teachings of yoga right into our everyday actions and reactions."

—ANGELA FARMER, cofounder of Yoga from the Inner Body

"This book is revolutionary! With great skill, Nischala Devi guides us on a journey through the Yoga Sutras; not through a dry, intellectual dissection of words, but by bringing us out of our heads and into our hearts, where the intuitive insights of these teachings reside. An inspiring guide that will nourish your practice and your life."

—JANICE GATES, author of *Yogini: The Power of Women in Yoga*

"By 'telling the story in another way' Nischala Joy Devi allows these ancient Sutras from the soul to resonate in your heart. She delivers a bounty of stories, examples, experiential exercises, and new ways to awaken sacredness and experience life as a living joy. Like a green coconut, *The Secret Power of Yoga* invites you to hold it in your hands and open it. Read each Sutra aloud; through Nischala Joy Devi's tender and subtle rendering may you find every line fresh, fragrant, and deeply satisfying."

—SHANTI SHANTI KAUR KHALSA, PhD, director of the Guru Ram Das Center for Medicine & Humanology

"Nischala Joy Devi illuminates a practical way to apply the Yoga Sutras to everyday living and spiritual awakening. Within the flow of her message is the trinity of *bhakti, jnana,* and karma. With *bhakti,* her approach and understanding come from the heart as she inquires into the heart of the matter. *Jnana* comes from her years of devotion to yoga. She complements this experience with cross-references to various classic scriptures. Karma is reflected at the completion of each sutra with a lesson that welcomes self-inquiry and calls for positive action. Nischala Joy Devi's commentaries, inspired from the feminine voice, will nurture many on the path of yoga."

—KALI RAY (SWAMINI KALIJI), internationally renowned yogini and founder of TriYoga®

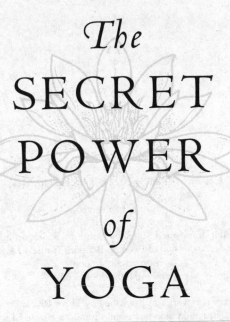

# The
# SECRET
# POWER
## of
# YOGA

*A Woman's Guide to the*
*Heart and Spirit of the Yoga Sutras*

NISCHALA JOY DEVI

Published in the United States by Harmony Books, an imprint of
Random House, a division of Penguin Random House LLC, New York.
HarmonyBooks.com
RandomHouseBooks.com

An earlier edition of this work was published by Three Rivers Press, an imprint of
Random House, a division of Penguin Random House LLC in 2007.

Harmony Books is a registered trademark, and the Circle colophon is a trademark
of Penguin Random House LLC.

Library of Congress Cataloging-in-Publication Data
Devi, Nischala Joy.
The secret power of yoga : a woman's guide to the heart
and spirit of the yoga sutra / Nischala Joy Devi.—1st ed.
1. Hatha yoga.   2. Exercise for women.   I. Title.   RA781.7D4854 2007
613.7'046—dc22                2006026162

ISBN 978-0-593-23556-0
Ebook ISBN 978-0-593-23573-7

Printed in the United States of America

Book design by Jo Anne Metsch
Cover design by Kathleen Lynch/Black Kat Design
Cover image by yotrak/iStock/Getty Images Plus

10  9  8  7  6  5  4  3  2  1

Revised Edition

ALSO BY NISCHALA JOY DEVI

*The Healing Path of Yoga*

*The Namaste Effect*

*Meditation in the Yoga Tradition*

To all the future generations of women and men

who will never even wonder if the

scriptures are also for women.

# CONTENTS

# THE WISE WOMAN'S STONE

A wise woman, who was traveling in the mountains, found a
precious stone in a stream.

She reverently placed the gem in her bag.

The next day, she met another traveler, who was hungry.

The wise woman opened her bag to share her food. The hungry
traveler saw the precious stone in the wise woman's bag,
admired it, and asked the wise woman to give it to him.

The wise woman did so without hesitation.

The traveler left, rejoicing in his good fortune.

He knew the jewel was worth enough to give him security for
the rest of his life.

But a few days later he came back, searching for the wise
woman.

When he found her, he returned the stone and said,

"I have been thinking. I know how valuable the stone is, but I
would like to exchange it in the hope that you can give me
something much more precious. If you can, teach me the
secrets about the power you have within you, the power that
enabled you to, without hesitation, give me this precious
stone."

# PREFACE

## THE WISDOM OF THE YOGA SUTRAS
## FOR PRACTICE AND LIBERATION

AS MUCH AS we would like life to travel at a steady and smooth pace, it seems to be in perpetual motion. The world continues to go through its gyrations; our lives seem to mimic or even exaggerate those changes. Some we welcome—others we would like to avoid. We often search for solutions to create a sense of steadiness, meaning, and calm to help us cope or even elevate us. Perhaps that path is Yoga.

Observing how Yoga has changed the world, I cannot help but wonder how the world has changed Yoga. As the plethora of Yoga studios and communities formed, they focused mainly on serving the physical body. The calling was great; strengthen and balance the body—that is what people knew, and that is where the need seemed to be the greatest. Many of the transformative physical benefits were touted, and the studios that sprang up were brimming to capacity.

While I held a great respect for and awe of the physical body, my real love was for the sacred wisdom teachings of Yoga. The connection to the inner teachings led me to wonder if those embracing Yoga *knew* the treasures hidden within the path they were treading. If they delved a bit deeper, they would reveal an approach more expansive than the mind could imagine. It fueled my intention to provide a more accessible pathway for any seeker who chose Yoga as set forth in the scriptures. Their reward would be not just a healthy and strong body but liberation itself.

With this inspiration, the first edition of *The Secret Power of Yoga* was born in 2007.

When I originally wrote this tome, I made certain choices and adaptations, hoping to make it accessible to many. The compromise in dealing with such a comprehensive sacred text was to translate and comment on the books I and II and summarize books III and IV. Books I and II are by tradition the most widely expounded upon and give even the most zealous student plenty to study and assimilate. They are the foundation of Yoga wisdom and practice, important for all serious students and teachers. At the time, I felt it was important not to overwhelm the student but rather to inspire and entice the seeker and encourage curiosity about the next steps. That was the correct decision, for then.

Books III and IV contain the most esoteric aspects of the Yoga Sutras, and because of this, they tend to be less accessible as the basis of a spiritual quest. They are expounded upon in the final half of the Yoga Sutras to deepen awareness as well as quench the thirst of the spiritual seeker as they reveal our essential nature. They are best understood and realized when the concepts explained in books I and II of the Yoga Sutras are intimately and thoroughly absorbed. Also, because of the more occult nature of these later sutras, it *seemed* a heart-centered perspective would not necessarily enhance their interpretation in the same way it does for the sutras in books I and II. But times have changed, people have changed, and Yoga has changed.

It would now be the exception to find a Yoga teacher or even student who has not had at least one course on the Yoga Sutras of Patanjali. With so many making a commitment to the practice of Yoga to further their own spiritual growth and development, it is time to offer the complete text.

Books I and II will always be the gold standard for describing the basis of Yoga. Venturing into books III and IV presumes that certain experiences and understandings explained in the earlier books have provided the foundation to build upon. Rather than assuming, "Oh, I already know the sutras. Let's go on," query, "If I continue to practice, what is in store for me?" It is a way of cajoling the mind to practice. As those of us faithful to daily practice can truthfully attest, it is not always exciting to sit and be still. Some days we may experience quiet, at other times restlessness. At a certain moment, when least expected, we realize the bliss the scriptures attest to.

Whatever the experience, we continue to practice.

This expanded edition of *The Secret Power of Yoga* unites all four books in one complete text, as was originally intended. Part I, "The Yoga Sutras: Its Wisdom and Practice," includes books I and II. The first part offers us wisdom to lead us in our daily lives and to kindle a deep quest to know the Self. It includes practices to encourage us on our way to realizing that resolve. Part II, "From Devoted Practice to Higher Consciousness," assumes a strong basis and foundation of practice as it propels us to the center of our spiritual reunion with ourselves. While the teachings may be far removed from daily life, we find ourselves on the doorstep of realization, and then we are gifted with realization itself. For some it may be too soon in their studies to venture into books III and IV, while others may feel encouraged to go deeper. Whatever the choice I place before you, it is here for the taking. My hope is that each person treading the sacred path of Yoga will find solace in these great teachings.

# A FOUNDATION
# FOR TRANSFORMATION

TODAY MILLIONS OF people practice the physical aspect of Yoga. Most of them are women. Why is this? Is it because we've read in magazines that Yoga will give us a better body, tighter abs, buns of steel, or that we'll look and stay younger? Or perhaps we come to Yoga with problems we need fixed: physical issues like stiff necks or sore backs, or emotional ones such as depression, insomnia, or anxiety.

If these are the reasons we initially attend class, what keeps us coming back to Yoga, even after our problems are resolved or we've gotten in shape? Does something happen deep within us after we have stretched and squeezed and twisted and bent? Is there a special feeling that comes when we let go for just a moment and experience something magical inside? Something that seems familiar, something we have longed for or forgotten? Perhaps touching that mysterious part of ourselves is so powerful that we're motivated to return to it again and again.

"The journey of a thousand miles begins with a single step," said the Chinese sage Lao-tzu. Now, for growing numbers of harried Americans, a single step into a Yoga class begins a transformative journey into the vast world that unites body, mind, and spirit. The physical part of Yoga practice has become a gateway to this ancient spiritual discipline. Once we cross that threshold, we open ourselves to limitless possibilities, and to realms many of us have yet to dream of. When we let go and look within, the power we experience can transform our lives.

*The Secret Power of Yoga* is the knowledge that lies on the other side of that threshold, the knowledge that we are not just our bodies, our minds, or our emotions. The *secret* that brings endless *power* is knowing that we are Divine Beings. This knowledge can permeate our entire lives, bathing us in peace, joy, and love.

## THE FEMININE FACE OF THE DIVINE

I'll never forget the opening scene from the movie *Yentl*, a tribute to women and their spiritual aspiration, directed by and starring Barbra Streisand. The narration begins with the line "In a time when the story belonged only to the men . . . ." Then we see a young, beautiful woman perusing the stalls of an open-air market in early-twentieth-century Poland. A lover of books and a clandestine scholar of the holy scriptures, she is attracted by a bookseller calling out to passersby, "Sacred books for men, storybooks for women. Sacred books for men, picture books for women."

She sneaks around to the men's side, where the sacred books are sold. "You're in the wrong place, missy. Sacred books are for men," the bookseller tells her smugly. "Is it written that women cannot read sacred books?" she asks, with a slightly rebellious tone. Condescendingly, he replies, "Do yourself a favor and buy a picture book. Women like novels." Realizing that she has no other recourse, she says, "What if I say it is for my father?" "Why did you not say so in the beginning?" asks the bookseller as he takes her money and gives her the book.

This story has always touched me deeply. As a woman who has taught Yoga for more than thirty years, I have felt a great deal of frustration, and at times sadness, at the fact that virtually all aspects of Yoga, from translations of sacred texts to instructions on performing postures, have been interpreted almost entirely by and for men.

I feel passionately that it is time for women to explore and validate the experiences they feel deep within, experiences that men could never articulate for them. We need to know that what we are experiencing is not unusual or odd but our true, unique, divine nature shining through. This knowledge must then be passed on to everyone, both women and men, empowering all of humanity with its gift.

As *Yentl's* story illustrates, it was not so long ago that women were not even allowed to read spiritual books, let alone provide commentary on them. Such prohibitions still exist in some cultures; women are forbidden to pray alongside men in many churches, mosques, and temples. Many religions draw strict lines between the sexes, laying out separate sets of commandments for women and men. Women may not be allowed to touch the holy books or even be in their presence. Those of us granted the privilege of reading the holy scriptures may notice that even in the great epics of thousands of pages, women are conspicuously absent in the text.

These traditions are so ingrained in our various cultures that we are often unaware of the patriarchal slant of doctrine and its consistent exclusion of women. The world has too long been viewed solely through male eyes. It is time for women to speak out and reinterpret the male-dominated scriptures in a way that resonates with our experience. And given the predominance of women practicing the physical aspect of Yoga, it seems natural to start with a woman's guide to the heart and spirit of the Yoga Sutras.

## EXTRAORDINARY POWERS, ORDINARY WOMEN

Among the hundreds of translations of the Yoga Sutras that exist today, almost all are written by men. Perhaps this is why so many of my female students have told me, "I have tried to read them, but they don't seem to relate to me. So I gave up. Can you recommend a translation that I can relate to?"

Until now, my answer had been no, because I, too, have found most translations unsatisfying or inaccessible. Yet it was not an easy decision to interpret the Yoga Sutras from my own experience and from a feminine perspective. I knew I would face controversy and disapproval. After all, as many have told me along the way, I'm not a Sanskrit scholar, a professor, or even an intellectual.

Yet our story as women is filled with seers, healers, and visionaries who formed an integral part of society, and most of them were not scholars or intellectuals. They were mostly unassuming women, living ordinary lives while exhibiting extraordinary powers. Their wisdom was derived from their very humility and open-mindedness. Very often, these women were tapping into their intuitive powers to heal or make awe-inspiring prophecies. Simple women reached into other dimensions as easily as stirring the soup or rocking the cradle, and in so doing they helped heal the sick and avert calamities.

Having this gift, this access to a higher order, was considered special but not unusual. These powers were once touted as "natural," something that all women could tap into. When viewed with an elevated consciousness, intuition was honored, not feared.

Tragically, this great and benevolent gift came to inspire fear. Women's intuition came to be regarded as "irrational" and women became second-class citizens. And in the darkest times many of the women exhibiting their intuitive powers suffered greatly at the hands of the ignorant. In the sixteenth and seventeenth centuries, countless women were tortured and burned alive as "witches," mostly in Europe and America. During these terrible times, most of those accused of having supernatural powers (which were often nothing more than the "power" of being beautiful) were women. Witch hunting *was* woman hunting.

Thankfully, most women in modern society are not treated as harshly as we once were, but prejudices still remain. We are tempted to hide our gifts for fear of physical, mental, or spiritual persecution. But the great stories of women tell us that concealing our power is detrimental to future generations. Truly and joyfully embracing our power honors the blessed gift it was meant to be.

## LANGUAGE OF THE HEART

The word "sutra" is related to the English word "suture," a thread that strings or sews things together. The Yoga Sutras weave together the warp and weft of our material and spiritual lives, creating an inspiring tapestry.

What many of us find lacking in the Yoga Sutras lies in its translations, written by and for male scholars from a left-brained, analytical perspective, often obliterating the wisdom it attempts to convey. It is my hope with this book to provide a unique commentary on the Yoga Sutras that emanates from the heart with an intuitive, feminine approach. Instead of translating the ancient Sanskrit to modern English, *The Secret Power of Yoga* reforms a variety of previous translations and interprets them in a new light, using "English of the heart," unlike the more conventional offerings that rely on "English of the mind."

Whenever a translation is offered, many of the prevailing prejudices, customs, and social standards of the time in which it was written are sifted into the mix. Since for a long time women were not highly regarded in a spiritual sense, the absence of emotionally centered parables and examples and heart-centered teachings can be understood. The hundreds of commentaries and translations of the sutras written by men only further the exclusion of women in the spiritual world. Studies have shown that when the pronouns "he" or "him" are written or spoken, people do not make the leap of recognition that this also includes "she" and "her." This is why we see a movement in contemporary writing toward alternating between "she" and "he" or, in some cases, using "s/he."

Originally, I chose to study and then to translate the Yoga Sutras as, unlike many of the sacred books, it presents a more gender-neutral approach. The original wording of the sutras, without commentary, rarely used specific reference to the masculine form. I felt as a woman I was welcomed there.

With many people now expressing a more fluid gender identity, we as a society need to find other pronouns that accommodate all beings, regardless of their gender preference. It is important that, reading the scriptures, we recognize ourselves in the sacred. Until we can formulate one or more pronouns that include all, the status quo will continue.

Having praised the Yoga Sutras for being gender neutral, imagine my surprise when I began to translate book IV, "*Kaivalya Pada: Supreme Liberation,*" the final and most occult aspect, and suddenly the masculine gender, including the pronoun "he," surfaced in the earlier translations. Originally, I did not expect that the final two books would be enhanced by a feminine, heart-centered perspective. Their descriptions seemed to be beyond any identification with the body, as the soul is without form or gender. But upon closer scrutiny of the translations of book IV, the gender-specific references abruptly returned.

The use of the pronoun "he" was resurrected, used not just personally but to define and reference *Purusha,* the True Self or godhead—then automatically deeming its counterpart, *Prakriti,* the force of nature, feminine, bestowing upon it the pronoun "she."

Is it necessary to characterize either aspect of the Divine as masculine or feminine? Both *Purusha* and *Prakriti,* used to describe spirit and nature, have existed since time immemorial. They appeared to have separate but equal importance. When embodied, these energies, inherent in all, were instilled in each individual as both *Purusha* and *Prakriti*. They were both designated equal and opposite roles within the same individual.

After a time, the origin of the equal and opposite was forgotten and the energies became polarized, leaving only the *established* fact that God is masculine. Myriad prejudices followed.

When masculine qualities are elevated and become the *only* representation of the Divine, either as *Purusha* or as any of the vast array of other masculine identifications of God, then *Prakriti,* as feminine, is by default given the lesser role and becomes, like any aspect of nature, something that needs to be controlled.

Instead of adhering to the gender misidentifications assigned to the godhead and to nature, we can create a more altruistic way to explain these two opposite and dynamic forces. Viewing this important concept through a different lens, we leave both the gender identification *and* the prejudices behind.

Drawing from natural phenomena, we know there are two equal and opposite forces that together provide balance and stability. The *centrifugal* force pulls and propels outward, while the *centripetal* force pulls and propels inward. It is understood that if one is present, both are present, and they are of equal yet opposite importance.

If we are able to align the forces of *Purusha* and *Prakriti* with this same understanding, opposite yet equal, spirit and nature would be envisioned as inner stillness and outward movement respectively. If this becomes the norm, the masculine and feminine principles will be understood as equal and opposite, as well as gender neutral.

Over the millennia, this gender misrepresentation has greatly influenced the denigration of women. Because of the perpetuation of this myth, women, girls, and nature were deemed inferior and, when not easily subjugated, were dominated and often enslaved.

With the passage of time the vastness of this concept was minimized and gender reference became the norm, leading the average person to identify themselves within the polarized stereotypes. Men became the *gods,* which relegated women to the role of *nature,* with the dubious honor of serving the gods.

This reference to God as "he" was further cemented throughout the holy books of varying faiths. The misidentification continues to flourish, even today, within various religious communities throughout the world. The great majority of time whenever the godhead is personified in human form, it is assigned masculine attributes and characteristics. Consequently, the supporting or secondary aspect is awarded to the feminine.

Even if the concept of an inward energy as equal and opposite to the outward-flowing energy is conceded, assimilating the concept into the established doctrine most religions adhere to is daunting. It would require the mostly male clergy and scholars presiding over the doctrine to be amenable to these modifications. Up till now this concept has been ignored and, in some cases, considered blasphemy, when in fact many of the scriptures declare that the indweller of the body, the spirit or divine self, is beyond all physical identification and form.

As the vast spiritual consciousness flows in the direction of oneness, the practical application of gender equality must keep in step. If not, the religions that cleave to out-of-date concepts will lose their moral compass, causing their followers to reject their spiritual guidance. Though clergy and scholars have been guiding society through the millennia, individuals will now be responsible for interpreting the sacred scriptures and teaching with their own hearts.

It is my intention in this commentary to neutralize the polarizing masculine and feminine. In some cases it is not possible to do this, as the identification and language are so ingrained and interwoven that the teachings would be confusing. When identification returns to the neutral, everyone gains the ability to see the Divine reflected in themselves. Once we have moved beyond all identification and are no longer bound by qualities of either feminine *or* masculine, *oneness* becomes the option.

In addition, our modern culture tends to separate and even polarize the heart and the head, feelings and thoughts. Feelings are often considered inappropriate, wrong, or even scary. Yet if we look closely at the teachings of many ancient cultures, they describe the heart, not the head, embracing both thoughts *and* feelings. To deny feelings and validate only thoughts denies the very essence of our being. For this reason, I have chosen to use the terms "consciousness" and "heart" where the customary translations would be "mind" and "thoughts."

In Hindi the word for "translation" means "telling the story in another way." *The Secret Power of Yoga* does precisely that, conveying the meaning of Yoga's most sacred teachings from a heart-centered, feminine viewpoint.

## DIFFERENT AGES FOR DIFFERENT CONSCIOUSNESSES

During ancient times, when the great spiritual scriptures were being formulated, the world was open to many kinds of interpretation. According to historical accounts, many early civilizations divided time according to eras of human development. Plato, the great Greek philosopher, described a cycle of 24,000 years called the Great Year, during which the consciousness of human society expands and diminishes according to certain cycles. In yogic philosophy, the same idea comes forth as four *yugas,* sequential time periods of civilization similar in concept to Plato's Great Year.

The *Sat Yuga,* or the Golden Age, was the first manifested era. In this time people's behavior reflected their pure consciousness and integrated it smoothly with their humanity. Righteousness was eternal. One's duty to be true to one's spiritual nature was foremost. There was no competition, disease, depression, or struggle. Fruits of the earth and heavens were obtained by imagining, by being openhearted, and according to personal necessity. This could also be considered a more inclusive, feminine way of being. It sounds like the utopian society that many of us dream about.

It was during this *Sat Yuga* that the Vedas were formulated. These great gems of wisdom were universal truths without reference to gender. They clearly proclaimed that *we are one*. And from the *Sat Yuga* of evolved consciousness came the next three *yugas*: *Treta,* or the Silver Age; *Dvapara,* the Bronze Age; and *Kali,* the Iron Age. In each successive age, virtue was further obscured and righteousness increasingly faltered.

Many believe we are now in or emerging from the *Kali Yuga,* the nadir of enlightenment, and there is plenty of evidence for that claim. Egocentric thinking, greed, and fear have become the norm. Our respect for Mother Earth and for feminine values has declined, contributing to an epidemic of anxiety, depression, and hopelessness about the future. Most of us consider it a luxury to take time to retreat from the outer world to the realm of the spirit, and it is promoted as a blessing for the chosen few. With all this comes a devaluation of love, faith, and other spiritual virtues, causing them to hide deep within our hearts. We place little value on spiritual qualities; instead, we worship the material.

The good news is that we proceed through the *yugas* in a circular progression. So if we are now emerging from the Iron Age, the *Kali Yuga,* we are coming back around toward the *Sat Yuga.* Because it has been many thousands of years since the time of elevated consciousness, little of that refined consciousness remains.

## UNLOCKING THE MYSTERY

The yogic path is the way to attain Golden Age consciousness. The Yoga Sutras, a great spiritual text and guide, embodies the purity of this dharma (righteous path). It weaves together a beautiful tapestry of essential wisdom and insights that allow us to know our divine nature. Much of this wisdom is distilled and simplified from earlier sacred texts: the Vedas, the Upanishads, the Bhagavad Gita, and perhaps some Buddhist texts. The Yoga Sutras uses the insights of these scriptures to depict the nature of consciousness and the path to liberation.

Though there is some uncertainty surrounding the origins of the 196 aphorisms in the text of the Yoga Sutras, historians have deduced that the sutras were originally compiled and codified by the great sage Sri Patanjali. It is thought that he lived at least 2,500 years ago. His aspiration (much like that of this book) was to restate these great teachings in a way that made them relevant to the people of his time. He also realized that if more people learned these great gems of wisdom, there was a greater likelihood that the essence of the teachings would be preserved and flourish.

The Yoga Sutras were transmitted orally and without commentary for a time before they were written down. When they were finally recorded in writing, they, like most other sacred texts, were engraved on leaves and then sprinkled with a colored powder so that the letters or characters could be read. The leaves were stacked rather than bound so that the teachings could be easily rearranged. The fixed arrangement in which we now most frequently see the Yoga Sutras is based on tradition.

*The Secret Power of Yoga*, while different in its interpretation, keeps the traditional format of most translated versions of the Yoga Sutras. It has four sections, books, or *padas*: book I, "*Samadhi Pada*: Union with the Divine Self"; book II, "*Sadhana Pada*: Cultivation of Spiritual Practice"; book III, "*Vibhuti Pada*: The Divine

Manifestation of Power"; and book IV, "*Kaivalya Pada*: Supreme Liberation." They are presented in their usual sequence and abide by the standard numbering.

This allows for easy study and the ability to compare a variety of different commentaries. Ideas and concepts are repeated in different parts of the text, helping to reinforce the importance of key teachings. This repetition is common in other great teachings as well, including the Bhagavad Gita and the Old and New Testaments of the Bible.

The creation of chapters happened as I was contemplating the presentation of this sacred text. It became apparent to me that many of the sutras were grouped together, representing the familiar venerable paths of *Bhakti Yoga* (devotion), *Karma Yoga* (service), *Jnana Yoga* (wisdom), *Hatha Yoga* (physical), and other categories. The Bhagavad Gita (one of the texts from which the wisdom in the Yoga Sutras was drawn) was the inspiration for presenting these aphorisms in chapters, as it, too, is presented in chapters.

I think it's a more manageable way to study the sutras, rather than the usual form of a long, continuous column; a smaller group of sutras can be studied and assimilated with relative ease. Also, this presentation suggests a variety of ways to interpret the repeated sutras, offering a different angle in each chapter. This system conforms to the traditional numbering system found in the Yoga Sutras.

The sutras themselves were written as partial sentences and sometimes seem to be thoughts or feelings hanging in the air. It is as if they were jotted down in note form, reminding the teacher what to say next. The Yoga Sutras as they were written allow us to question and interpret them and relate them to our particular situation and life. The eloquent pearls of wisdom are strung together to form one of the most concise, elegant, and complete teachings of Yoga available today.

Scholars and pundits East and West have translated and re-translated the Yoga Sutras, but most of the original translations from Sanskrit to English were done by a few Western scholars living in British-ruled India. Their hope was to shed some light on these great threads of wisdom as they made them available to the English-speaking population. These translators brought with them education, clarity, and experience, along with their prejudices and cultural differences.

Western religious traditions differ from Eastern traditions in numerous ways. The fundamental understanding of Eastern wisdom is that divinity is granted by birth, whereas in the Western traditions divinity is usually something to continually strive for, and only a select few realize it, through grace or by their own accomplishments.

The mysteriousness and oddness that Western translators observed in the Indian culture caused them to cling even more to their familiar philosophies. This lack of understanding of the culture greatly influenced their translations. It is difficult, even now, for the *Western mind* to understand the complexities and subtleties of an *Eastern mind-heart*. The puzzle piece that seems to be missing is that, in Indian society, the *heart and feelings are fundamental to, not separate from, life*. This basic concept is the essence of Eastern sacred prayers and scriptures.

## THE GOLDEN AGE OF LEARNING BY HEART

We have all had the experience of learning something by rote to pass a test. Often we call this learning "by heart." How many of us can remember this material now? But that which is truly learned by heart is never forgotten. The secret power of Yoga can be found not by intellectual reading or discourse alone but by deeply meditating on each aphorism, imbibing the spiritual truths and bringing them to our everyday life.

This way of learning may seem an unusual practice for our

modern times, yet it is how spiritual teachings have been transmitted in Eastern culture from ancient Vedic times to the present. This learning process has three parts: *Sravana* (listening), *Manaana* (reflecting), and *Nididhyasana* (experiencing). Often a teacher would recite a sutra without explanation or commentary. The student would then retreat to reflect on the "feeling" the sutra evoked, thereby uncovering its meaning. After some days, weeks, or months the student would return to the teacher and a discussion of a deep and profound nature would occur. The students were literally taking the teachings to heart.

*The Secret Power of Yoga* is oriented in this way. First the sutra is presented for silent and spoken repetition: You are encouraged to *listen,* understand, and feel the sutra. The commentary that follows invites you to *reflect* on the wisdom of the sutra using stories, parables, and personal insights to further instill the heartfelt meaning. The all-important *experiencing,* which is usually absent from the more traditional Yoga Sutra texts, is then proposed so the essence of each sutra can be integrated into everyday life.

## THOUGHT AND FEELING

Sanskrit, the language of the sutras, is particularly well suited to this heart-centered approach because it is a vibrational language, one in which words resonate through countless layers of meaning. When this powerful vibrational language is translated literally into a very logical and straightforward language like English, many of its subtleties may be lost. The strength of the English language lies in precise, concrete explanations. It is less powerful when describing the subtler realms, the unity of the feminine and masculine, and especially the intuitive realm.

Before we begin to formulate a word or even a thought, a feeling is experienced that stems from a vibration. This vibration that triggers the feeling is then translated into a thought, a thought to a

word, a word to writing, a complex process that happens in a heartbeat. When we read, the word is connected to a thought, which
then traces back to a feeling or a sensation. It happens so quickly
and often that we fail to notice that each thought is the outgrowth
of a feeling.

We see this phenomenon echoed in the formation of our physical bodies: The heart forms much before the brain. The process
begins with the joining of the egg and sperm, then the process
of replication produces undifferentiated cells. Within a few short
weeks of embryonic development, the cells begin to differentiate,
and with those first specialized cells a tiny heart is formed. This
early formation of the heart allows us as new beings to be guided
by the rhythm of the spirit, and it is from the heart that feelings are
born, flowing through us into each cell.

The brain, thought to be the provider of thoughts, develops
much later than the heart. The heart remains independent in its
rhythm until near the time of birth, when the central nervous system takes over the regulation of the heart. From then on, the heart
is reliant on the brain, and subsequently feelings seem to combine
with thoughts and the two become virtually indistinguishable.

Yet when we feel something deeply, our ability to convey our
experience in words lessens. Enraptured by the beauty of a magnificent sunset, our thoughts are stilled. We may find ourselves
explaining to others, "Words can't describe such a deep feeling."
Given the extraordinary difficulty of putting transformational feelings or divinity into words, it's easy to understand why rational
thinking became dominant. We then superimpose the organiza-
tional structure of the physical world onto the spiritual realm, for
lack of an adequately delicate design. Trying to express the subtle
in mundane terms, we are perplexed. For this reason, the *Nididhyasana* (experiencing) aspect of the study of the sutras can be the
most vital. By honoring our feelings and the intuitive places of our

being, we create the deep union between the heart and the soul. We can then spark the remembrance of who we *really* are, not just mirror the physical reality.

> True spiritual success is never gained through mere reading of books.
> —*Yoga-Shastra*

## SPIRIT OF THE SUTRAS

For many years I've been a student of the Yoga Sutras. I've sought to understand them from a "rational" view. This striving relaxed as the "heart perspective" invited itself into my study. Embracing the *spirit* of the sutras, rather than their literal meaning, allows me to integrate the sacred teachings at a much deeper level. In a way, it is like bypassing the mind and going directly to the heart and the soul. This allowed me to "feel" the vibration of what is meant.

As I am not a Sanskrit scholar, I have included only the few key Sanskrit words from these ancient texts, those that are most familiar. If this kindles your interest for more of the original language, there are scores of books and a few great teachers on the subject. The way I have chosen to share these great teachings with you is to reach into my heart, feel what wisdom they are imparting, and share that with you.

In *The Secret Power of Yoga* the negative words that are found in the English language in abundance have been excluded where possible in order to bring a more positive vision to this sacred text. This was a difficult task, considering the English language has the habit of taking a negative word and adding a "not" or an "un-" to it, expecting the opposite meaning to emerge. But in actuality, the mind continues to relate to the root word, and we miss the important concept. For instance, the great virtue *Ashteya* in the Yoga Sutras is typically translated as "nonstealing." Upon hearing this, the mind cannot help but focus on "stealing"—exactly what we've been told not to do! For an opposite effect to take place, the word or words must be reinterpreted from "what not to do" into "what to do." *Ashteya,* then, could easily be understood in positive terms such as "honesty," "generosity," or "integrity." So rather than implying that people steal and proposing they refrain from this action, this text will propose that they be generous and honest and live in integrity.

Similarly, the sutra on *Aparigraha* is generally translated as "nongreed" or "greedlessness." Telling someone not to be greedy is like telling them not to think of chocolate. Once the notion of chocolate is planted in the mind, it's very hard to dislodge. A more positive approach goes to the heart of *Aparigraha* and unveils the positive perspective as "awareness of abundance," so that sharing what you have and taking only what you need follow naturally.

This same concept is often seen when words from other languages are adapted. Their literal meaning gives way to what they imply. For example, when they are put together, the French words *chaise* (chair) and *longue* (long) come to mean more than a long chair. "I am going to sit in the chaise longue" implies that this type of chair affords comfort and relaxation. We may then adapt the spelling to more easily fit into English, as we have with "lounge chair." Here the meaning of the word *longue* (lounge) changes from "long" to "relaxation," describing its *effect* rather than what it *actually* is.

## OFFERING THIS WISDOM FROM THE HEART

As a young yogini, I was on my way back from co-leading a weekend retreat when my mentor, the swami in charge, informed me he would be leaving the ashram permanently in two days! My response was total shock. Ignoring my reaction, he continued, "I am in the third week of an eight-week Yoga Sutra course."

"What will happen to the class?" I asked naïvely. With a smile he reached into his briefcase, handed me a copy of Patanjali's Yoga Sutras, and said, "Start studying!"

The night of the first class I taught, I was very nervous. What would people expect? What did *I* know about the sutras? What if I gave them incorrect information? At the time, there were very few translations available in English. The preferred way to learn the sutras was from a living teacher, one who taught as well as lived the wisdom. Still very young, I did not feel I had spent enough time sitting at my master's feet, absorbing the sutras in my own life. Certainly I was not steeped enough to teach others.

What was I to do? I did the only thing I knew how to do: pray. I prayed and prayed and prayed again. With that sincerity, my heart opened, and I experienced the inner wisdom of the sutras. My sense of clarity was restored. I now understood that knowledge received from an open heart transforms intellectual understanding.

My hope is that what I have presented here is useful, understandable, and in keeping with the truths of the Yoga Sutras. If they resonate with how you feel, take the teachings into your heart and make them your own. Meditate on them; use them in your life. Most important, remember the feeling of empowerment, the knowing that all of us, women and men alike, no matter how we may appear or sometimes act, are *Divine Beings* in human form.

Each of us holds some Golden Age consciousness within us, and it is ripening right now. The more we begin to acknowledge our inner spirituality and let it shine, the more we let heart and spirit reign supreme, the sooner we can make the Golden Age a reality.

From my heart to yours, I hope you enjoy the journey to discovering *The Secret Power of Yoga*.

Nischala Joy Devi

*The*

# SECRET
# POWER
## *of*
# YOGA

# A JOURNEY THROUGH
# THE SUTRAS

*Seek not to learn the sutras.*
*Instead seek to learn who is the one*
*who studies the scripture.*

In "A Journey Through the Sutras," each sutra presented is numbered and in sequential order according to the traditional form. They are commented on individually or in clusters that have similar intentions or that when joined together complete a significant idea. This same clustering may also be applied to the section on *experiencing* at the end of each commentary.

The format of the sutras that follow supports the three stages or ancient ways of imparting knowledge described earlier: *Sravana* (listening), *Manaana* (reflecting), and *Nididhyasana* (experiencing).

The first stage, *Sravana* (listening), is facilitated by saying the sutra aloud, without the commentary. This aspect of listening is so vital, it is presented in three different ways at various places in the text. The first place you will encounter *Sravana* is in the list of complementary sutras at the beginning of each chapter. When repeated aloud in sequence, the rhythm of the words leads us to an understanding greater than each one could elicit individually. It presents the chapter's wisdom at the level of vibration.

You then meet each sutra individually before the actual commentary. Because you will have recited them at the beginning of the chapter, you will already be familiar with them. Take a moment to draw in a deep breath and, with wholehearted awareness, repeat the sutra or sutras aloud as you *listen* to the great teaching reverberating through your body, mind, emotions, and spirit. The opportunity to repeat this ritual will appear frequently throughout the commentary of each sutra. Each time it does, stop and *listen* to what the sutra is telling you. Allow the wisdom to be imparted before going on. In this way you will access the deeper, more intuitive form of knowing.

*Manaana* (reflecting) is the stage that elicits a response from both rational thoughts and heartfelt feelings. This is accomplished through the traditional wisdom, stories, parables, and personal insights found within the commentary of the sutras. The intention is to satisfy the great spectrum of wonder, revealing a fuller understanding. As much as possible, relate this section to your life and circumstances. It will spark your heart's desire for knowledge.

*Nididhyasana* (experiencing) assimilates the earnestness gained from *Sravana* with the understanding gained from *Manaana,* unfolding the timeless truth of each sacred gem. These practices derive from the practical essence of each sutra. They enrich our perception by bringing us closer to the truth, often bypassing the questioning and rational mind. The *experiencing* often outshines any reluctance to change our previous ways.

PART I

# THE YOGA SUTRAS:

*Its Wisdom and Practices*

# BOOK I

## SAMADHI PADA:

*Union with the Divine Self*

&

# BOOK II

## SADHANA PADA:

*Cultivation of Spiritual Practice*

*Whether you are a beginner or a continuing student of the Yoga Sutras, a whole new way of viewing yourself, others, and the world awaits you.*

*That statement in a curious way is a caution. When you begin this journey, many beliefs and previous ways of being will come into challenge; it may even contradict the way you live your daily life.*

*Studying the sutras over time will invoke a yearning to know yourself, your true self. Altering the way we live our lives can either enhance inspiration or diminish this yearning, causing it to hide in the shadows.*

*As you explore these sacred teachings, new ideas will surface. Some you will instantly embrace, while others may seem distant, foreign. Acknowledge the contrast, welcome the new ideas. Give yourself the gift of time to decide which to pursue or discard.*

*Books I and II give us a glimpse into the sacred ways of Yoga, revealing who we are in the highest sense. They establish our perception that when consciousness unites, our birthright as a Divine Being is revealed. To the delight of many, this supreme wisdom is enhanced by an abundance of practices, allowing the wisdom gained to be experienced.*

*Many of us, while enjoying the bounties of the material world, are eager to have a foothold in the spiritual as well. A time will come when our spiritual being will seductively beckon, and we will willingly obey. For many it will come after we have exhausted every effort to satisfy our wants and desires in the material world.*

# BOOK I

# SAMADHI PADA

## *Union with the Divine Self*

Book I, "Samadhi Pada: *Union with the Divine Self,*" offers generous insights into those parts of our being seldom visited and establishes the perception that when consciousness unites, we know we are Divine Beings.

Here Samadhi Pada carefully and methodically reveals guidance to explain how our lives would differ if we believed we are at once both human and divine. It brings to light the simple fact that if we nurture only one aspect of our being, the other will withdraw.

It is time to recognize that when our humanity is in harmony with our divinity, every moment, thought, emotion, or action is infused with spiritual essence.

# HUMBLE BEGINNINGS

*With humility (an open heart and mind),*
*we embrace the sacred study of Yoga.*

## I.I *With humility (an open heart and mind), we embrace the sacred study of Yoga.*

This simple beginning holds many truths. Often this very first sutra is read quickly or even disregarded, which is unfortunate since this sutra is placed first to set the tone. It is here to remind us that our study and spiritual path benefit most when they are paved generously with humility.

## DEVELOPING AN OPEN HEART AND MIND

As students of life, we often need to look at where we have come from to see where we are going. I was always enthralled by the subway in Paris. At each station a giant board helps you find your way. A little arrow indicates where you are, and with the push of a button you select your destination. As the destination registers—voilà!—a path lights up the most efficient way to get there. Wouldn't it be wonderful if our life path were that clear and simple?

Our present position has been determined by the past—all those crossroads where we made decisions, each path we've taken that brought us to our life as it is. We might be able to understand how we got where we are, but what would it have been like if other options had been followed? Another choice could have radically changed the present. Perhaps we took the tried-and-true course because it seemed easiest, or safest; perhaps at the time, it just didn't seem like there was any alternative.

> What you are is what you have been.
> What you will be is what you do now.
> —*Lord Buddha*

Occasionally we meet someone who took an uncharted route, one less established. What in her life led her to become a trailblazer? What inspired her to leave behind the beaten path? The found path may have brought great adventures or great peril. Most of us are content to know that our future will be spiced with a few obstacles and sprinkled with safe adventures. Very few of us want to risk our comfort.

Custom and tradition play a major part in shaping our lives. We are so embedded in them that unless we are repeatedly shown a different way, we tend to live out our days under their sway. "We always have yams for Christmas. Why do you want to change tradition this year and have mashed white potatoes?" This tendency toward inaction and stasis can be difficult to overcome. But being creative and trying something different can be exciting and can expand your horizons. If it is carried beyond what is understood, it can cause rejection. Not wanting to offend, we may choose to reject the "new" idea that might have brought us renewed happiness and expansion.

Most of us in modern societies are very blessed. We are literate and have books as resources. Sacred texts can be downloaded from the internet. But even though they are so easily accessible, it is important to have the same regard and reverence for these sacred teachings as in times before.

One of the key teachings of Yoga which we will find sprinkled throughout the sutras are the *gunas*. From this understanding we can adjust our habits to calm any interference with our spiritual growth and ultimate liberation.

## THREE GUNAS (ASPECTS OF NATURE), TEACHERS OF HUMILITY

As students of spirituality, our yearning for the truth varies in intensity. Some of us may fit in a few spiritual practices at our convenience; others may dedicate their entire lives to their spiritual unfolding. Born with certain tendencies called the *trigunas,* or three attributes of nature, we are part of nature and are perpetually influenced by her.

This wisdom is drawn from the Chandogya Upanishad. It explains that all of nature, people included, contains an uneven mixture of the three gunas. One of the characteristics is always dominant. (See more on the gunas in sutra 1.16, page 57.)

*Sattwa* is best translated as a sense of balance. *Rajas* is reflected in activity and overactivity, taking things to the extreme, while *Tamas* is inactivity, or being withdrawn, and can lead to difficulty focusing and acting, or inertia. The world and everything in it constantly moves between these three states, varying from minute to minute, day to day. This can be seen in the growth of a flower: *Tamas* is the plant in seed form, and *Rajas* is the growth action needed to bring about fruition. Once it has bloomed fully, intense action decreases, giving way to being, and *Sattwa* is present in the pristine flower blossom.

It is not possible to move directly from *Tamas* to *Sattwa,* although they may appear the same from the outside. To go from *Tamas* (inactivity) to *Sattwa* (balance), movement or *Rajas* (action) must be traversed. From that movement dynamic stillness comes, as *Sattwa.*

At night, as the natural light wanes, we become more indrawn and quieter (*Tamas*). During the day, when the light is strong, we tend to be outward and active (*Rajas*). At the two moments when day and night blend delicately together, at dusk and at dawn, there is balance (*Sattwa*). This quality is the reason dawn and dusk are observed in many traditions as auspicious times for prayer and meditation, times of special equanimity.

In South India, a beautiful custom honors these three aspects of nature. When approaching a spiritual teacher for the first time, a prospective student offers the teacher a whole green coconut. (There, green coconuts grow on trees, a whole version of the ones we find here in supermarkets.) For the offering to be meaningful, the tree must be climbed and the coconut cut down. Then, according to tradition, the student has the arduous task of removing the tough green husk with a machete. This is a vital process, analogous to preparing the student's mind and heart for the teachings, to remove resistance or qualities of *Tamas*.

This process exposes the inflexible and brittle nature of the nut's hard brown shell. It represents the *Rajasic* part of our ego that is strong and thinks it knows everything. The coconut is then humbly presented to the teacher, or guru—a fitting name that means "one who removes darkness or ignorance, so that we may see the light of truth." With discrimination and deep compassion, the guru breaks open the hard brown shell of the coconut. The lily-white inner sweetmeat is revealed, symbolizing our *Sattwic* nature.

**With humility (an open heart and mind), we embrace the sacred study of Yoga.**

## EXPERIENCING THE DIVINE IN EVERYTHING

*Sit quietly and light a candle if you wish.*

*Begin to make a mental note of your daily activities. How much of your day do you spend on simple, repetitive chores that do not feel immediately rewarding? Do you sometimes feel they are a waste of time?*

*Begin by focusing on one of these activities, such as making the bed each morning. How can that be transformed into a spiritual practice?*

*Can you savor the smooth feeling of the linens? Can you have fun plumping the pillows? Put in some happy vibrations and feelings, so that when you get into bed at night, you will have happy dreams and a deep sleep.*

*Next you might turn to the routine of checking voicemail, answering calls, filing papers, paying bills, washing dishes, or picking up your children from school.*

*Notice how each aspect of your life can be inwardly transformed to bring you to a place of presence and joy. There we recognize that the Divine is omnipresent.*

# WE ARE *ALL* DIVINE

THE following sutras enlighten us as to who we really are and how we experience life when we are in that state of knowing. They also remind us that as our consciousness moves outward, we separate from our essential nature. It is this identification with our Divine Self that leads us to joy.

*Yoga is the uniting of consciousness in the heart.*

*United in the heart, consciousness is steadied, then we abide in our true nature—joy.*

*At other times, we identify with the rays of consciousness, which fluctuate and encourage our perceived suffering.*

## 1.2 *Yoga is the uniting of consciousness in the heart.*

*Yogah Chitta Vritti Nirodahah* is the Sanskrit transliteration of this well-known sutra. Through this one sutra we are able to know the true essence of Yoga.

Deep within our hearts, we abide as pure Divine Consciousness. But with the material world pulling us every which way, our consciousness is drawn outward. As our knowledge of the Divine Self slowly fades, it takes with it the understanding of our true nature.

*Chit* is pure universal consciousness and *chitta* is the same consciousness individually expressed. *Chit* is the ocean of consciousness, vast and unlimited. At birth each of us gathers a small quantity of this vastness and encases it in the temple of our heart as *chitta*, individual consciousness. Held for many years, it remains unchanged. Then, at the end of our life, it is released back into the ocean of consciousness; the recognition of oneness causes the *chitta* to instantaneously unite with the *chit*.

Many translations of the Yoga Sutras link this sutra to notions of controlling one's mind and thoughts. Trying to gather and control the multitude of thoughts and emotions with no knowledge of their origin is a daunting idea and a very difficult task.

It seems to be a compromised way of explaining the concept of consciousness to a culture that does not have roots in the belief that we are *all* divine.

Consciousness abides in the heart, not in the mind, as many believe. But when we realize that it is the *heart* that is the holder of our consciousness, reunion—once understood to be a difficult task—seems more likely.

When this sutra is translated referencing only the mind, the emphasis is on control, restraint, or some form of restriction. It encourages students to be harsh with the consciousness. But the heart responds more readily to tenderness, and gentle, caring treatment of your consciousness is the best way to liberate it.

Notice your hand gestures when you are speaking to someone about who you are. Gesturing to my heart when I say "I am Nischala Devi" reveals the truth: "I live right here in my heart."

**Yoga is the uniting of consciousness in the heart.**

## YOGA WITH A CAPITAL Y

Today the word "Yoga" conjures up the image of some difficult or contorted pose. Once relegated to a few faraway ashrams or caves, it is now practiced in gyms, health clubs, and studios all over the Western world.

What is being taught under the name of Yoga is a minute part of this great tradition, a microscopic focus on the physical. Yoga in its completeness is a way of life that allows for total transformation. But the physical postures, or asanas, can serve as an introduction to this distinguished wisdom tradition. Asanas reintroduce us to our bodies. Once we become friends with the physical, going inward to the spiritual becomes easier. Yoga in its completeness is a way of life that allows for total transformation.

## AND THE BODY LEADS US

My early experience with Yoga, just like that of most Yoga students today, was mainly physical. Not a very physical person by nature, I nonetheless endured all the stretching and bending, hoping to find something more.

I brought my search into yet another Yoga class, this time at the Integral Yoga Institute in San Francisco. As soon as I walked in the door, I was struck by a photo of the teacher beaming at me, face aglow with love and compassion. Somewhere inside I knew that Sri Swami Satchidanandaji, whom I later discovered to be an exalted Yoga master, was the teacher who would ignite my soul, guiding me on my inner journey back to my own spirit. Integral Yoga enabled me to balance body, mind, and emotions, reminding me that through opening my heart I could touch the depth of my soul. Yoga became one of the greatest blessings of my life.

Yoga takes us back to the beginning of our journey of becoming human; we spark the memory that we are first and always an aspect of the Divine. The physical body was created as a temple to house this divine light.

One starry night our mother and father felt that spark, and before long, the largest and smallest human cells, egg and sperm, were united. We were on our way to a physical birth; our temple was being built. Our mission, as we were already divine by nature, was to integrate our divinity with our humanity. No striving for divinity, no original sin, only the recognition of our true nature.

Born helpless into the physical world, our tiny being is over-whelmed by sensory stimulation. Finding the confines of the human body excruciatingly restrictive, we spend most of our time traveling in the astral world, brought back to earth only when the body needs food or a soiled diaper replaced, or when we are called back by the love of others on earth.

As time goes on, we spend more time in the physical body, and the processes of thinking and feeling begin to mature and occupy more of our consciousness. When at last we fully settle into the body, the challenge is to remember that we are divine, as well as human, beings.

This is the essence of this sutra: to remember that we are, and always will be, Divine Beings who have become divinely human. Divine Consciousness emanates from our hearts, infusing our bodies, minds, emotions, and very lives.

*Yoga is the uniting of consciousness in the heart.*

When we are able to realize this truth, all the sutras that follow *Yogah Chitta Vritti Nirodahah* are unnecessary. For most of us,
however, the study of *all* the sutras is a necessary reminder, as we
are quick to forget who we *really* are. As we embrace each subsequent sutra, we hope to uncover that which is obscuring this truth
and come closer to living by it.

When delving into Yoga, it is up to you to choose how you image
yourself *and* others. It is important to remember that *you are not
the only one who is divine.* Everyone is the same as you, just housed
in different containers, shapes, and temples, embracing the same
essence. Your relationship with the Divine Consciousness deepens or lessens according to your observance and treatment of yourself *and* others. Divine Being *or* human being? Divine Being *and*
human being? Your choice.

The more we cloak our divinity, the dimmer the spark becomes.
If we choose to shape our lives according to the lesser amount of
light, rather than the boundless amount of light from the source, this
becomes the yardstick by which all our experiences are measured.

*Yoga is the uniting of consciousness in the heart.*


## AS SERENE AS A MOUNTAIN LAKE

Imagine consciousness in all its purity as a clear mountain lake.
Gazing into the lake, we can see the mirror image of the mountains that surround it. This pristine illumination mirrors our divine
nature. While all is still and calm, the mind and heart rest in their
divine nature, and we experience love and oneness for all.

A gentle wind blows across the lake, and the clear images become slightly wavy. The crystal clear reflection of the light is

disturbed, yet the distorted image can still be seen. If the wind continues to strengthen, the reflection of the mountains is soon completely obliterated.

The wind represents our thoughts and emotions, at first gentle and then strengthening. As the wind increases, it stirs up the bottom of the lake, and the clarity of the reflection is replaced by muddy turbulence. It may happen occasionally at first; and then slowly, without our realizing it, it becomes more and more frequent. Eventually, our divine nature is no longer being luminously reflected.

After some time, this motion causes the shore to wash into the lake, forming sandbars. Our thoughts and feelings form these clusters of habitual patterns, tendencies, and potentialities, called *Samskaras*. The *Samskaras* accrue by the constant churning of the thoughts and emotions. Whenever any thought or feeling encounters the wind, it is easily fed into one of these patterns. Then our habits and tendencies become set and the mountains disappear from view. The pattern of habit, or *Samskara*, is difficult to change, as our consciousness is often unable to reconfigure the obvious. An unexpected change in circumstances can be missed, if we look only for the predicted course. Once the sandbars have developed, it takes a great wind of change to modify their shape.

### Yoga is the uniting of consciousness in the heart.

The lotus flower has long been a symbol for the unfolding of spirituality. It is one of the most elegant illustrations of the meshing of our human and divine natures.

The lotus seed is planted and grows in muddy waters, below the surface of the lake, far from the light. Though the light is murky and unclear, the flower blossoms by drawing energy from within. As the bud passes through the muddy waters, it lifts its face to the sunlight and finally emerges. Miraculously, not a trace of soil remains on the flower. It lives in the mud yet is unaffected by it. This is an example for us to be in the world but not be adversely affected by it. The lotus flower teaches us that no matter how muddied the waters of our consciousness may become, clarity can always emerge from our spirit if the Divine Light guides us—even if it is only one tiny lotus blossom at a time.

> I looked in temples, churches, and mosques.
> I found the Divine in my heart.
>
> —*Rumi*

*Yogah Chitta Vritti Nirodahah.*
*Yoga is the uniting of consciousness in the heart.*

## EXPERIENCING THE DIVINE SPIRIT WITHIN

*In a softly lit room, sit as close as comfortably possible to a mirror.*

*Take a few deep breaths in and let them out slowly.*

*Allow yourself to relax.*

*Take a moment to look at your own familiar face.*

*Allow thoughts to drift away. Bring the awareness to your eyes.*

*Keep your eyes soft as you gaze deeply into them.*

*At first you may feel uncomfortable. (We rarely, if ever, look ourselves in the eye.) But the eyes are the windows to the soul, so take a look into your own.*

*Continue to relax and soften the gaze.*

*Find yourself going deeper within until you get a glimpse of the Divine Light that is ever present.*

*Repeat either silently or aloud, "I am a Divine Being."*

*Start by doing this for one minute, and build to five minutes or more.*

*As you allow your eyes to close, be still and experience any feelings that surface.*

*What did you experience? Could you feel the depth of consciousness within?*

*Practice two times a day for one week and observe how your newfound feelings and thoughts influence the vision of your true nature and other people's as well.*

*Each time you pass a mirror or think of yourself in any way, reaffirm, "I am a Divine Being."*

## 1.3 *United in the heart, consciousness is steadied, then we abide in our true nature—joy.*

When consciousness reunites and remains undisturbed, our true divine nature is revealed as joy. The expression of this joy is infinite love, which encompasses and then transforms everything it touches. Everywhere we look, we see the reflection of our divine and joyful nature.

Many of us have had a glimmer of this feeling when we are falling in love. Everything looks brighter; even gloomy days cannot dissuade us from our bliss. We radiate joy and greet the world with openness and clarity. People smile at us, mirroring this loving energy back to us. This then serves to remind us of who we truly are, and the glorious cycle continues.

Recently, I was in the midst of making some very complicated travel arrangements. My flight schedule was a particularly important missing piece, so I called the airline. As usual, I was quickly put on hold while some dreadful Muzak filled my ear. Every so often a mechanical voice assured me that my call was very important to the company. As the minutes ticked away, I believed it less and less.

Finally, an agent came on the line. It was, I admit, a complicated flight arrangement, but the length of time it took him to do it did not match the job. I was losing my patience. Using my idle pen while I was awaiting the schedule details, I began to write "Om Shanti," the peace mantra, to regain my calm. Periodically he would come back to let me know that he was "still working on it." I thanked him and went back to my meditative writing.

Quite a while later, he came back, very apologetic that it had taken so much longer than he had hoped (me too!). We *finally* finished the arrangements and I thanked him.

"I want to thank *you*," he said.

"Why would you want to thank *me*?"

"This has been one of the worst days of my life. Ever since I came in this morning, each call I received got progressively more abusive. I know I'm not quick, but I try to do my work diligently. But people have just been so impatient today. At two minutes to five I was writing up my resignation. Something told me to take one more call. It was you. You were so kind and patient and, well, loving to me. Even though I was slow, you weren't harsh to me. I was able to remember that I'm a good worker. Because of your kindness, I have decided not to quit. I pray that I may have many more customers like you. And for the ones that are not, I pray to have your patience."

I was amazed. It was as if he felt the vibration of the *Om Shanti* mantra, which enabled me to be so patient. Love is the common thread that unites us. When consciousness is united in the heart, the reality manifests, and we know that we are all one in joy and love.

*United in the heart, consciousness is steadied, then we abide in our true nature—joy.*

## 1.4 *At other times, we identify with the rays of consciousness, which fluctuate and encourage our perceived suffering.*

Identifying with murky thoughts and feelings is like looking in a distorted mirror or a muddied lake. Those unclear images are often reinforced by the outside world. When we identify with grumpy or angry thoughts, the mind beams them outward. Similar thoughts and similar people are attracted to us as if magnetically. When we feel sad or fearful, friends who feel the same may call us. After all, misery loves company!

As we come to understand that our nature is joy and love, perceived suffering is unable to take root. Realizing that we do not have to be bound by any one interpretation, we alter our mode of identification. We then recognize and relate to our highest consciousness.

Imagine yourself standing in front of an enormous structure, one so large that it does not appear to have any boundaries. It is adorned with so many images, sayings, and words that the vastness keeps you engrossed. Even if at times the writings and images are disturbing, you remain attentive. Finally glancing around for a moment, you spot a small opening, not much larger than your eye. You never imagined this structure had any kind of depth. Its surface seemed so complete and all-encompassing.

Pressing your forehead to the wall, you peer through the small opening and are instantly transported to another reality, an incredibly beautiful scene filled with radiant light and glorious color. The disturbing images and messages that seemed so real only moments ago evaporate, like rain touched by the sun's radiance as it emerges from the clouds. You are transported through the portal to a peaceful vision. Once you taste the joy of living in beauty and love, you no longer find anything captivating about suffering.

## KISS THE OTHER CHEEK

I was at Dulles International Airport accompanying Mataji Indra Devi, one of my beloved teachers (then ninety-five years young), to her departing flight. Since saying goodbye to her students was always a lengthy process, she was running a bit late, so we sped to security, tossing her carry-on bags onto the conveyor belt. As she was about to walk through the metal detector, Mataji turned around and walked the other way!

"Oh no, what's she up to now?" I thought, conscious of the seconds ticking away. Oblivious to the movement of time, she had spotted an obviously unhappy security guard, whom I had sped by without noticing. She headed back toward him. Fully five feet tall in shoes, Mataji planted herself directly in front of the towering six-foot-five-inch guard. Standing on tiptoes, she reached up and took hold of his necktie. Using both hands as if climbing a rope, she pulled him down so that they were face to face. Stunned, he did not resist. I was aghast. What would happen? Would she be arrested? Should I try to stop her?

Mataji let go of his necktie with one hand and placed the other behind his head, and then planted a big kiss right on his cheek, complete with a loud smacking sound. Releasing both his tie and him, she turned and walked away. The guard was reeling, a smile of amazement on his face. She then casually walked through the metal detector, and, addressing my obviously surprised look, shrugged and said, "He needed that." As if that explained everything!

We are missing much joy if we allow the world to dictate the direction of our thoughts and feelings. But when our heart guides the focus of our consciousness, love is ever present in our life.

*At other times, we identify with the rays of consciousness, which fluctuate and encourage our perceived suffering.*

### EXPERIENCING YOUR TRUE NATURE AS LOVE

*Find a quiet place to either sit or lie comfortably.*

*Take in a few life-affirming breaths, and let them out easily.*

*Gently bring the awareness to your heart center, the seat of consciousness.*

*Observe as the consciousness is drawn away from the heart, attracted by any discomfort in the body. It could be your leg or arm, or a cramp in your back or neck.*

*Gently gather the consciousness and draw it back to the heart.*

*Repeat silently or aloud, "Yoga is the uniting of consciousness in the heart. I abide in my own true nature—joy."*

*Again observe as consciousness is drawn from the heart, attracted this time by the mind and its myriad thoughts.*

*Gently gather the consciousness and lovingly return it to the heart.*

*Repeat silently or aloud, "Yoga is the uniting of consciousness in the heart. I abide in my own true nature—joy."*

*Observe the movement of consciousness from the heart toward emotions and feelings.*

*Gently gather the consciousness and lovingly return it to your heart.*

*Repeat silently or aloud, "Yoga is the uniting of consciousness in the heart. I abide in my own true nature—joy."*

*Gently repeat this sutra anytime you notice consciousness moving away from the heart. It will aid you in bringing it back to your heart.*

*Slowly take in a few deep breaths. Notice how joyful you feel, living from the heart.*

*It is helpful to practice this for at least ten minutes each day and to repeat frequently throughout the day the sutra "Yoga is the uniting of consciousness in the heart. I abide in my own true nature—joy."*

# CHAPTER 3

# RAYS OF CONSCIOUSNESS

C ONSCIOUSNESS expands outward from the heart as we become part of the physical world. This cluster of sutras enables us to understand how consciousness ventures from its home in the heart and manifests as emotion and thought. The degree of clarity to which it manifests forms the framework for our life.

*Dividing into five, these rays of consciousness polarize as pleasant or unpleasant.*

*The rays manifest as knowledge, misunderstanding, imagination, deep sleep, and memory.*

*Knowledge embraces personal experience, inference, and insights from the wise.*

*Misunderstanding comes when perception is unclear or tinted.*

*Imagination is kindled by hearing words, seeing images, or experiencing feelings.*

*Deep sleep allows us to withdraw from conscious awareness.*

*Memory is when a previous experience returns to conscious awareness.*

## 1.5 *Dividing into five, these rays of consciousness polarize as pleasant or unpleasant.*

Our thoughts and feelings are trained by habit to flow in predictable patterns, which determine whether our life fosters a sense of ease and happiness or turns from it. These patterns are so ingrained that even the hint of a possible directional change is incomprehensible. Constant identification with these patterns forms our belief system, a blueprint for our lives.

Many belief systems seem to hold that difficulty is beneficial, and growth comes only with pain. This is reinforced by the all-too-popular adage "No pain, no gain."

Perhaps we should reconsider this philosophy. A small measure of discomfort *may* be necessary to encourage growth, but how much? Our hearts hold the hope that growth can be gained through love and kindness.

After a complicated dental procedure, I was given a prescription for pain medication. "Thank you," I said, returning the slip to the dentist. "I don't take any medication."

"You might want to rethink that. Research has determined that when even moderate pain is experienced, the healing process is inhibited," my dentist said, returning the prescription to me.

Could this same phenomenon be experienced on other levels, too? What if instead of hoping for pain to bring rewards, we simply turned directly to the rewards themselves? We may not have the ability to determine the outcome of every situation. We can, however, choose how it affects us, by looking at it from another view. Often I refer to those unpleasant times as the "cosmic itch," which presents just enough discomfort to keep me from getting too complacent yet not enough to cause real difficulty.

Whichever belief system you subscribe to, know that you possess the power to affect your life's patterns and dreams. When a thought, feeling, or situation arises, it will naturally flow into the groove that presents the path of least resistance. Which beliefs present that avenue for you?

Imagine if they were like those of a dear friend of mine. "How are you?" I asked her, on seeing her for the first time in a long while. "I am in my usual state of grace," she replied. "The difference is, this time *I know it!*"

We are all in a constant state of grace, yet how often do we remember?

*Dividing into five, these rays of consciousness polarize as pleasant or unpleasant.*

## EXPERIENCING HOW YOUR BELIEF SYSTEM INFLUENCES YOUR LIFE

*What is your belief system? Do you feel closer to the Divine when you are in crisis or in joy?*

*Do you invite hard times because you believe that they will help you to become stronger?*

*Notice how you have set up your life to foster those beliefs. Are you happy with your choice?*

*Pick one particular feeling, thought, or phrase that you use frequently. It could be "Life is hard" or "Life is good."*

*Actually count how many times you use it in a day. How does the meaning influence your day and ultimately your life?*

*Only you have the power to change your life.*

## 1.6 *The rays manifest as knowledge, misunderstanding, imagination, deep sleep, and memory.*

When consciousness ventures from its center, it forms rays that take on diverse characteristics and intents. With clarity and a keen sense of observation, these rays can be understood as distinct aspects of the one consciousness.

*The rays manifest as knowledge, misunderstanding, imagination, deep sleep, and memory.*

## 1.7 *Knowledge embraces personal experience, inference, and insights from the wise.*

The first ray of consciousness is *knowledge,* which then divides into three distinct aspects. These three aspects of knowledge illuminate the other rays of consciousness.

### CAN YOU RELY ON PERSONAL EXPERIENCE?

The first aspect of knowledge is personal experience. Where does this come from? The senses gather information from the sense organs, which is then interpreted by the mind and emotions.

When this information resonates with our bodies, minds, and emotions, a clear and identifiable knowing is confirmed. Living from that place, the whole universe seems to make sense. Knowledge becomes a steady, reliable friend.

But it is not always so amicable. If the mind and instruments of perception are murky, our perception becomes tainted or false.

Our mind and senses can trick us. At the scene of an accident, for instance, if there are four witnesses, then there are at least that many versions of what happened. How could that be? It was the same event viewed by people with the same sense organs who saw it with their own eyes and heard it with their own ears.

The organs of the senses are not faulty; it is our individual perceptions that distort. As a scene is filtered through thoughts and feelings, past experiences and prejudices, it becomes different for each person. Until they shine with perfect clarity, take your personal experiences with an ounce of caution.

*Knowledge embraces personal experience, inference, and insights from the wise.*

## IDENTIFYING INFERENCE

The second aspect of knowledge is inference. Often we experience knowledge from a deep place that carries no apparent reasoning. We honor this as our intuition. It is a sense of knowing that may have no other explanation or experience to reinforce it. It stands in its own power.

Inference, however, based on lucid perceptions can also help us to discriminate and to make decisions.

Seeing a cow give milk, we may then infer that all cows give milk. We confidently believe that if we can find a cow, we'll find milk. Only with careful scrutiny can we observe the difference between a cow and a bull. Without discrimination, inference might encourage us to attempt to milk a bull, putting us in peril with not a drop of milk to be had.

This aspect of knowledge can be very precarious. Many prejudices perpetuated by inference are taken to be the truth. Hearing about an individual from a minority race, religion, or national origin who has committed a crime, many find a temptation to lump all people "like that" together as criminals. If someone in a fancy sports car cuts you off on the highway, you might find yourself thinking harsh thoughts about the wealthy.

Instead of these judgments, use your power of inference to give people the benefit of the positive. Making gross generalizations places people in opposition, and what we do to others we do to ourselves. Look for the good in all things and all people. Hone your skills of discrimination and keep your heart open when you initiate inference. And always honor your intuition!

*Knowledge embraces personal experience, inference, and insights from the wise.*

## RECOGNIZING THE WISE

This aspect allows us to acquire knowledge through the wisdom of others that is often based on their own deep understanding or experience.

For many, knowledge is legitimized when it is written or spoken by an expert or a prophet. We consult the holy books (Bible, Koran, Vedas, Yoga Sutras, Gitas, etc.). Traditionally forward-thinking scientists or intuitive clergy boldly analyzed and interpreted formulas or passages, often challenging their peers. When they were able to prove their theories "correct," these theories became truth. We then embrace these "truths" as our touchstone. For some of us, therefore, knowledge must be accompanied by a deep resonance within.

At the time when the scriptures were formulated, very few common people were literate. Before the time of written scriptures, most of the teachings were orally transmitted, often to a congregation; for the especially devout, they were conveyed directly from teacher to student. When the direct transference of wisdom was accomplished, any doubts were alleviated. In those times of oral tradition, minds and emotions were sharper and less cluttered. The spoken word went deeply and directly to the heart.

As the scriptures were committed to writing, they underwent a continual process of evolution, modification, revision, and translation. This was accomplished by a small group of men who were privileged enough to have a high level of education. Often segments were lost, truths omitted, and stories reinterpreted. It is often difficult for women to accept many of the scriptural concepts as truth because of their inherent prejudices against the sacred feminine. Miraculously, there are still a cherished few of these writings that ring out with a truth that resounds with women. It is up to us, however, to find the flowers among the weeds.

The greatest wisdom is the insights experienced in our own hearts. This is the wisdom we cannot deny. The more we trust and honor it, the more it guides us.

> All truths are easy to understand once they are discovered;
> the point is to discover them.
>
> —Galileo Galilei

*Knowledge embraces personal experience, inference, and insights from the wise.*

## EXPERIENCING THE THREE WAYS
## OF KNOWLEDGE

*Choose a concept or a passage from a great spiritual book. Or choose anything else that inspires you.*

*While reading, observe if it resonates with your heart. Do you feel harmonious with the basic concept? Are there some aspects of it that you resonate with more than others?*

*Search until you find a passage or a commentary that supports your feeling.*

*If one does not reach you precisely, reword, rearrange, or broaden the idea until you feel in accord. This allows the passage to be more inclusive and sing to your heart.*

*When you hear its song, you are experiencing true knowledge.*

## 1.8 *Misunderstanding comes when perception is unclear or tinted.*

*Misunderstanding*, the second ray of consciousness, is a common fluctuation that may cause us a great deal of unpleasantness. Often we assume with certainty that our minds and emotions correctly interpret our sensory input, but do they? Many longtime resentments are perpetuated due to misunderstanding. Family members may hold grudges for years, and even take them to their graves. Often the next generation is unaware of the feelings of bitterness they inherited from their relatives.

Listen carefully with heart and mind, and ask for clarification when there is even the slightest doubt. And most important, use a liberal amount of forgiveness for mistakes—after all, the mistake might be yours.

*Misunderstanding comes when perception is unclear or tinted.*

### EXPERIENCING WAYS TO CLARIFY UNDERSTANDING

*Recall a recent time when you were involved in a misunderstanding. It could have been important or trivial. Is it clear to you where the misunderstanding occurred?*

*Go through the whole scenario again from the beginning, and bring clarity where it was absent before. Try to smile at the way things were misconstrued. Imagine the outcome to be comfortable for all concerned.*

*When there is a misunderstanding, can you forgive even if you were inconvenienced or put in an uncomfortable situation?*

*Can you forgive even if you are right?*

*Would you rather be right or happy?*

## 1.9 *Imagination is kindled by hearing words, seeing images, or experiencing feelings.*

*Imagination* is the third ray of consciousness. When it is illuminated, it becomes the path leading us to and from our heart's center. Imagination allows us to create an unlimited number of both pleasant and unpleasant experiences. An image is felt, and from that a thought, a word, or an action sprouts. When it is bathed in negative imagination, the image can have an unsettling effect. For instance, worry is the most prevalent form of imagination for many people. And all of us have been frightened by something that appeared to be there, only to later discover that it was not a threat to us or our loved ones. Do you easily reach for the worst-case scenario? When the imagination goes so far out, it takes immense effort to bring the mind and the emotions back to calm.

Perhaps taking a pleasant stroll to the mailbox, you find an unpleasant surprise: a letter from the IRS. Likely your whole body goes into a stress response, terrified that you are being audited or owe money. In an instant you are trying to figure out where you can borrow the money. The envelope is not even opened yet! Holding your breath, you open it—and an instant smile of happiness travels from your face to your whole body. It is a refund, and a big one at that! Worry and negative imagination led you to anticipate the worst. Such an immediate and transforming reaction affecting the whole body is one of the reasons imagination and imagery have become very powerful tools for healing. A positive image can elevate us and support us to heal. The opposite can cause many physiological systems to malfunction and cause disease.

*Imagination is kindled by hearing words, seeing images, or experiencing feelings.*

## TAKING THE TIME TO DAYDREAM

Daydreaming is another form of imagination. Although it is usually thought to be a waste of time, science is now finding that it actually provides a mini vacation. I was always scolded in school for daydreaming and wasting time. Who would have thought that I would now teach that very skill to people to help them heal! Every great individual—thinker, artist, musician, gardener, cook, mother, or anyone else—uses imagination as a way of setting the creative process in motion. What looks like a daydream is in fact your most productive moment. It is in your power to formulate pleasant *or* unpleasant experiences.

> Imagination is more important than knowledge.
>
> —*Albert Einstein*

*Imagination is kindled by hearing words, seeing images, or experiencing feelings.*

## EXPERIENCING YOUR CREATIVE, POSITIVE IMAGINATION

*How keen is your imagination? Do you imagine the absolute best for yourself?*

*Write down your hopes and dreams as an affirmation to help solidify them on the physical plane.*

*Your imagination is infinite; use it lavishly to the smallest detail.*

*If you are experiencing a physical or emotional imbalance, use your imagination to create the affirmation that will allow you to see yourself whole and healthy.*

*Engage all of your senses as part of the affirmation. The more real it seems to you, the more likely it is to become real.*

*Each day recite and experience your affirmation as it enhances the new image you have created of yourself.*

*Practice this with any and all aspects of your life.*

## 1.10 *Deep sleep allows us to withdraw from conscious awareness.*

*Deep sleep* allows us to withdraw from conscious awareness, offering us the luxury of temporarily forgetting. It is like having a holiday from thoughts, emotions, worries, and cares by completely letting go. Sleep is necessary for health and balance, providing a time for the body to repair itself and for the mind and emotions to release.

If we are to function effectively and lovingly during the waking hours, the deep sleep that allows us to rest in our inner consciousness is of prime importance. When we are well rested, our spiritual practices harmoniously unite all aspects of our being, allowing us to know who we really are.

> That we are not much sicker and much madder than we are is
> due exclusively to that most blessed and blessing of all natural
> graces, sleep.
>
> —Aldous Huxley

*Deep sleep allows us to withdraw from conscious awareness.*

### EXPERIENCING THE EFFECTS OF DEEP SLEEP

*Can you observe the effects of a good night's sleep on your body? Your mind? Your emotions?*

*Notice how you feel after a deep, dreamless sleep. Refreshed and rejuvenated?*

*Notice how you feel after a fitful night of dreaming and waking. Tired and perhaps a bit cranky?*

*Can you relate how you slept to what you watched, read, discussed, or ate the night before?*

*What was engaging your consciousness during that time of deep sleep? You may not be able to know exactly what happened during sleep to your body, mind, or emotions, but both the positive and injurious results can be felt.*

*Observe how your sleep pattern affects your life.*

## 1.11 *Memory is when a previous experience returns to conscious awareness.*

All day long, year after year, we take in impressions, which are then filed and stored within us. We are actually made up of volumes of memories that then create our present and future. We choose which memories are kept ready and available in the forefront—and which are tucked away in the unconscious. Our concepts and ideas need to be carefully weeded and released on a regular basis so that our consciousness can keep evolving. Without this constant vigilance, we find we live with stored memories that anchor us in the past.

Repressing unpleasant memories, though, can lead to serious problems. Although dormant, unpleasant memories can be triggered at very inopportune moments, causing us to relive the discomfort they brought us. A word of casual conversation with a friend may conjure up a memory of betrayal or abuse. This triggers feelings from the past that come flooding back, overwhelming present emotions. Misplaced hurt or anger may encourage an argument. Later, when trying to understand what happened, you may realize that it had less to do with your friend than with a long-forgotten memory relived.

On the other side, if pleasant memories are deeply planted, they may have the ability to encourage an easeful feeling even if life's woes are ever present. A situation may present itself in which you would have felt uncomfortable or threatened, yet recalling the pleasant memory radiates a feeling of peace.

The yogic practices help us release memories without having to express them either outwardly or in dreams. They also help dissolve unwanted thoughts and feelings as they are forming, relieving the need to see them to fruition or preserve them for a later time.

Sometimes while you are sitting still in meditation or holding an asana (pose), a memory will escape from the bottom of the mental-emotional lake. Like a bubble, it will float through layers of the subconscious and then pop on the surface of the conscious mind. It then becomes your choice to keep it or let it go. By bringing them up at a time of peace and relaxation, you can control your memories, rather than letting them control you.

*Memory is when a previous experience returns to conscious awareness.*

## EXPERIENCING THE RETURN OF MEMORIES

*Bring a memory of your choosing back to consciousness.*

*Notice what kind of physical sensations and emotions come with it.*

*Are you able to separate the memory from the sensations? Or are they one and the same?*

*Try to find its origin inside your body.*

*Then try gently to release the memory.*

*How does the experience of release feel?*

# PRACTICE AND REMEMBER

HERE we are given the key to balance and the way of power that aids us in our quest for the True Self.

*Consciousness is elevated by* Abhyasa *(devoted practice) and* Vairagya *(remembering the Self).*

*Devoted practice,* Abhyasa, *cultivates the unfolding of consciousness.*

Abhyasa *is nurtured by a sustained, steady rhythm and a dedicated heart.*

*With constant remembrance of the Self,* Vairagya, *all yearnings fade.*

*When consciousness unites, it remains clear and unaffected by the external changes of nature, the* gunas.

*This is the ultimate* Vairagya.

*By cultivation of* Abhyasa *and* Vairagya, *the intellect becomes keen, reasoning is clear, bliss is reflected to all, and outward identification unites with the Supreme Consciousness.*

*With continued awareness, we identify only with the pure consciousness residing in the heart.*

*Through identification with pure consciousness, the physical
world can be transcended.*

*This identification is enhanced by faith, dynamism, intention,
reflection, and perception.*

*To the dedicated and devoted, the divine truth is revealed.*

*Spiritual consciousness develops in direct proportion to one's
dedication.*

## I.12 *Consciousness is elevated by* Abhyasa *(devoted practice) and* Vairagya *(remembering the Self).*

Here are two necessary components to reunite us with our True Self. Imagine that *Abhyasa* (devoted practice) and *Vairagya* (remembering the Self) are two wings of the same bird. They are companions in play as they flap in unison, enabling the bird to fly: When they are seemingly still, the bird glides. Moving into a change of position, one wing lowers and the other raises. This complementary movement allows the bird to fly with grace and ease. Rhythm is the secret to the bird retaining its elevation; for us, rhythm keeps our consciousness elevated.

When a devoted practice is cultivated, that inspires us to remember the Self. This balances and brings grace to our daily rhythm. As we remember the Self, the effects of our simplest actions are considered. We relinquish old mindless habits (*Samskaras*) by intentionally choosing what to invite into our bodies, minds, hearts, and lives. "If I eat this large meal late at night," you might ask yourself, "will I be able to wake up early and be alert for *Sadhana* [spiritual practice]?" The correlation between eating a big meal in the evening and feeling light and alert in the morning becomes clear.

It takes time and patience to cultivate such understanding. At first opting for immediate gratification, we may toss all consequences to the wind and indulge in that large meal at night. The lethargy of the next morning encourages us to have a deeper consideration the next time a similar situation presents itself. With this new awareness, we are able to evaluate both the immediate and long-term effects of our decisions.

In order to soar, the bird needs both wings to flap to the same rhythm. When in balance, both wings are strengthened. Whatever challenges are encountered, with *Abhyasa* and *Vairagya,* we embody the skill and assurance to ride the currents.

*Consciousness is elevated by* Abhyasa *(devoted practice) and* Vairagya *(remembering the Self).*

## 1.13 *Devoted practice,* Abhyasa, *cultivates the unfolding of consciousness.*

To continually elevate consciousness, it is necessary to cultivate *Abhyasa*—devoted spiritual practice. As we develop a deep friendship with our inner Self, the fluctuations of thoughts and feelings recede and the comfort of the truth unfolds. Our senses and the material world constantly pull us outward, away from our inner consciousness. With deepening devotion we are encouraged to rediscover that divine spark within. It then becomes our first choice of identification in any given situation.

*Devoted practice,* Abhyasa, *cultivates the unfolding of consciousness.*

## 1.14 Abhyasa *is nurtured by a sustained, steady rhythm and a dedicated heart.*

Here we are given three ways to nourish and deepen a methodical spiritual practice. What exactly is a devoted practice? What does it mean to nurture our practice by a sustained, steady rhythm? And for how long? A month? A year? Ten years? It is not possible to have a formula to determine something as acutely personal to each individual.

Often students will become frustrated. "I've been practicing meditation for three months now, and I still don't feel anything different."

"What is it," I ask, "that you expect to feel?"

"I don't quite know, but I expected something otherworldly to happen," they answer.

Even if we do not realize it, what we are seeking is the sense of wholeness. This sense is so familiar that often we forget that it is always with us. The time we spend each day in communion with ourselves is such an integral part of our lives that when it is absent, we feel unbalanced and out of sorts. Rhythm of practice, on the other hand, can be one of the most stabilizing effects of our life.

The rhythm of a devoted practice is sustained and steady when you no longer have to ask, "Should I sit for meditation today?" Now there is no need to make excuses, to look for a reason to take a day off. A Benedictine monk who devoted himself to spiritual practices for more than thirty years once told me that if for one moment he hesitated or questioned, he would have left his vocation. Observing his deep inward smile, it was obvious what he would have missed.

**Abhyasa** *is nurtured by a sustained, steady rhythm and a* *dedicated heart.*

## WHOLEHEARTED DEDICATION DEVELOPS A WHOLE HEART

In order to sustain a dedicated heart, choose a practice that encompasses the richness of spirit in everyday life, one that nourishes you on all levels. If you are devotional by nature, tend toward chanting or other practices that complement the heart-centered feeling. If you are more intellectual by nature, you might be attracted to the study of holy scriptures. The predominantly physical person might

enjoy the more active asanas (poses). But for the most harmonious effect, try to create a well-rounded balance in your choice of
practices.

Simple repetition is not enough for true *Abhyasa*. Our practice
may be as steady as a drumbeat, yet to fully embrace the spirit of the
activity, a deepening must take place. A metronome beats a steady
rhythm, but it is the heart of the musician that imbues the music
with spirit and life. This kind of transformation takes place when
our practices, traditions, and teachers are wholeheartedly honored.

In time most daily rituals—cooking, driving, eating, giving
someone a kiss goodbye, even meditating or engaging in spiritual
practice—can become rote or routine. Keeping the enthusiasm
alive is the key. After months or years of doing the same poses,
breathing techniques, and chants, the heart may lose its hold on
the practice. Don't discard them; instead, rededicate your heart to
them. Lavished with love, they can be transformed into a practice
that resonates for you. The striving then stops as the heart takes
over. The ordinary is transformed into the extraordinary!

> The secret of genius is to carry the spirit of the child into old age,
> which means never losing your enthusiasm.
>
> —*Aldous Huxley*

**Abhyasa** *is nurtured by a sustained, steady rhythm and a
dedicated heart.*

## EXPERIENCING THE RHYTHM OF YOUR
## SPIRITUAL PRACTICE

*What is the rhythm of your practice?*

*Is it steady like a metronome?*

*Is the rhythm too fast or too slow? Regular or irregular?*

*Is there anything you can add to enhance your heart's participation in the practice?*

*Introduce flowers, a plant, a beautiful mat, a pillow, or a photo of nature or of an exalted being into your sacred place.*

*Do whatever you can to encourage the union with the Divine Self.*

## 1.15 *With constant remembrance of the Self,* Vairagya, *all yearnings fade.*

As our focus turns toward "remembering the True Self," we naturally identify less and less with external desires or wants. This perspective reveals that we are merely the temporary caretakers of whatever we possess. With this attitude, nothing binds us. As life bestows gifts upon us, we are delighted. With their revocation, we may feel momentarily upset, but with the grace of remembering our Divine Self, our emotional equilibrium is quickly restored.

Through remembering the Self, or *Vairagya,* we become lucid and vibrant like a diamond. Millions of years of pressure on a simple lump of solid coal transforms it into a pure, transparent diamond that reflects and refracts light. This prismatic effect showers rainbows of colors on everything without discrimination (*viveka*). The diamond also appears to take the color of any object nearby. But once removed, it is perfectly colorless again. Likewise, when our minds and hearts clearly reflect our true nature, we may acquire many things, but nothing permanently taints our clarity.

With this lucidity, we enthusiastically adopt that which enhances the light, and redirect that which dims it. As we become free, we become more and more comfortable with the natural flow of material things. Much of what we yearn for comes to us. We enjoy the treasures of the world while they are with us, knowing full well we will not bind to them, nor they to us. And as they depart, our arms open wide and let them fly. Steady in both circumstances, we remember who we really are.

This concept has its greatest challenge when we are separated from our friends and loved ones, especially without our permission or when it seems permanent. Our heart feels a vast emptiness where it was once filled with love. At these times it takes great strength to restore and sustain our equilibrium. By securing a place within our hearts to hold their love and by continuing our devoted practice, our balance is more easily reestablished.

**With constant remembrance of the Self,** Vairagya, *all yearnings fade.*

## CAN WE BE ATTACHED TO NONATTACHMENT?

Often *Vairagya* is explained as "nonattachment." This is a harsh misunderstanding that promotes avoidance of a situation or a person, based on translations that guide us toward what not to do, instead of what to do. This interpretation of *Vairagya* grants permission to be cold and uncaring, "nonattached," as a way of not getting hurt by others or negatively attached. Such a stance is often accompanied by a large dose of fear and insecurity. It is exactly the opposite of the oneness our hearts are leading us to.

Similarly, we may find ourselves separating from some of the sweetness of life for the sake of being "spiritual." Many people associate spirituality with being withdrawn and even a bit cranky. This, too, is a misconception. We are at once divine *and* human; spirit dances together with nature, and its expression is joy!

*With constant remembrance of the Self,* Vairagya, *all yearnings fade.*

What about those yearnings? Where do they all come from? How do they embed themselves so deeply in our thoughts and emotions? As newborns, we are in a constant state of *Vairagya,* easily remembering ourselves as Divine Light. Our purity and innocence projects a wide-eyed, openhearted sense of wonder. At the same time we experience an exquisite feeling of helplessness. Bathing, eating, dressing, moving our bodies, the most basic of care, is beyond our capacity. Yet we hold no judgments about the world and neither accept nor reject the world's image of us. Slowly, we become more independent and are able to explore the world. We begin to understand criticism and find we are shrouded in judgments for such simple acts as soiling our diapers or dribbling when we eat our food. Our instruction book of do's and don'ts has begun to be written.

"Blue is for boys, pink is for girls."
"Girls play with dolls, boys play with trucks."
"People who come from this place are bad and steal."
"Only this school is good."

Confusion begins to occur at that young age, since we are still so closely identified with our divine nature. Are we not in fact Divine Beings, and isn't everyone else also? Do I need to trade this divine reality for earthly consciousness? Will this new set of rules eventually become my main reflection?

Our family and teachers continue to instill guidelines in us based on their own social understandings and prejudices. They feel it is their duty to do so, out of love for us and the desire to prepare us to live in society. Unfortunately, through the millennia, rules have taken precedence over love. As we internalize more traditions and social codes, we are forced into the lifelong balancing act of weighing our divinity against respect for society's rules.

## THREE CHARACTERISTICS OF INDIVIDUAL CONSCIOUSNESS (*CHITTA*)

Through all these conditionings, the universal consciousness, or *chit,* remains the same. But as our material awareness flourishes, it begins to recede from us. The consciousness we retain is individual consciousness, or *chitta,* which is differentiated into three features: *buddhi, manas,* and *ahamkara.*

*Buddhi* functions as intellect and intuition, *manas* refers to sense perception, and *ahamkara* is the ego self-perceiving itself as a separate entity. Their cooperation allows us to reason, to perceive the world, to function, and to grow according to our individual needs.

The *buddhi,* as the discriminative and intuitive aspect, has no likes or dislikes. It stores information and then relays it to the *manas* (senses) or to the *ahamkara* (ego-self). It harmoniously resonates with our inner knowing. The *buddhi* wants and needs nothing for itself and is experienced as a clear reflection of consciousness. (The name Buddha, meaning "the enlightened one," is derived from the word *buddhi.*) The *manas* functions as a receptor of sensory data. Our sight, hearing, taste, touch, and smell are governed by the *manas.* Unable to discriminate on its own, it feeds the sensory information back to the *buddhi* for clarification and validation, or to the *ahamkara* for action.

The *ahamkara* is the sense of "I, me, mine" that is commonly called the ego. This is the part that receives information from the *manas* (senses) and the *buddhi* (discrimination). It either desires or rejects their findings. "I want that" or "I don't want that." The ego has a poor reputation in spiritual circles as the part of our individual consciousness that divides and separates rather than unifies. In fact, we need a healthy ego to function in the physical world. When the ego is vibrant, it guides us to reflect our true nature, allowing the inner and outer worlds to flow together in harmony.

Perhaps, as you are walking down the street one fine day, you are feeling exceptionally content and in harmony with your surroundings. The *manas* begins to pick up a signal from the organ of sense—in this case, the nose—that a delicious smell is in the air. The smell begins to entice the sense of taste, causing your mouth to salivate. This alerts the *buddhi,* which then searches to identify the smell. "The odor is cinnamon, often used in cakes and pastries," the *buddhi* reports.

As your sensory involvement mounts, the eyes now engage with the words on a nearby window. The *buddhi* recognizes the word "bakery." Now the vision, smell, and taste are involved in the discovery. The eyes spot a small, round spiral with little particles on top that appear sticky. The information is inputted and comes back identified as a "sticky bun with nuts."

Also stored in the *buddhi* is the resolve that you are not going to eat sugar for the next couple of weeks. Meanwhile the *ahamkara* (ego-self) has been enjoying the day and not paying much attention to what was going on, but with the perception of the sticky bun, it jumps into action. "Sticky bun?" The words suddenly summon its attention. "Where are there sticky buns?" Connecting immediately with the senses (*manas*) and ignoring the *buddhi* (discrimination), it informs the legs to march into the bakery. The hands seize a sticky bun and the *ahamkara* instructs the mouth to bite and chew it, finishing the tasty delight within seconds! Content once again, the *ahamkara* renews the resolve to not eat sugar. This time it will have less power because it was so easily ignored. As we can see, all three aspects work together. The greatest influence will come from the one aspect of the three that has been strengthened and respected the most. If you allow discrimination and intuition to officiate, rather than trying only to satisfy your ego and senses, greater contentment will be the fruit.

But sometimes you may choose to override reason and follow your desires, as in the example above. Don't then feel guilty about your decision or agonize about how bad it is for you. This ruins the enjoyment of the moment and encourages negative effects on your health. Guilt *opposes* spiritual growth. If you make the decision to eat something you decided previously to avoid, then completely enjoy it! It is the ego that wanted it, but now the ego is not letting you enjoy it! Instead, trick the ego and enjoy the experience.

Regret and guilt are just different forms of yearning—the yearning for the past, the yearning for another chance at a decision. Instead, remember yourself, and remember that you followed your own choice.

**With constant remembrance of the Self, Vairagya, *all yearnings fade.***

### EXPERIENCING REMEMBERING THE SELF, *VAIRAGYA*

*Make a list of what is important to you. People first, things next. Could the people and things on your list continue to be well cared for if you held the constant awareness that you are a Divine Being? By making this remembering a top priority, could you give even better care and love to others?*

*Maybe you and a friend are in a restaurant and you are insisting that she order your favorite dish. Consider how your mind and emotions react as you are subsequently told that there is only one portion available. Your friend instantly says, "You have it; I can easily order something else." Do you insist that she have the dish, or do you feel it is "yours"?*

*If that situation is too easy, try something more challenging. What type of reaction do you think you would have if you found out that someone less qualified than you received "your" promotion?*

*Or if the person you really hoped would invite you to the biggest event of the year took someone else?*

*Observe how you react to the many daily events in your own life.*

*As the remembrance that you are divine takes deeper root in your consciousness, challenges may test your conviction.*

*Make sure to remember your True Self in all conditions!*

1.16 *When consciousness unites, it remains clear and unaffected by the external changes of nature, the* gunas. *This is the ultimate* Vairagya.

The more we remember the Divine Self, the more brightly the pure diamond light is reflected. Resting in that light, we are unaffected by external changes.

We again are called to look at the interplay of the three attributes of nature, or *gunas: Tamas* (inactivity), *Rajas* (overactivity), and *Sattwa* (balance), which we spoke about in sutra 1.1. The world and everything in it constantly moves among these three states, but if we are able to remember the Self at all times, they are unable to influence us.

All nature, including us, reflects this continuous cyclic movement of time and change. The relentless play of the *gunas* is like waves crashing onto the shore and then rushing to merge back with the sea. It is often called the Sea of Samsara (the sea of birth and death). Helplessly caught in this illusion of tumultuous changes, we experience valuable lessons here on earth. As we long for steadiness and balance, we observe and then transcend the constant movement that inhibits us from reuniting with our essential nature.

## OUR MINDS AND EMOTIONS COME IN TECHNICOLOR

When we identify with the *gunas* (rather than the True Self), the clear light within becomes prismatic, showering a rainbow of colors (*varnas*) on the mind and emotions. This rainbow literally colors how we think and feel, and these colors are reflected in our common parlance.

*Tamas,* a state of inactivity, manifests itself most extremely as an inability to make decisions, or immobilizes us through fatigue or fear. A positive attribute of *Tamas* is its ability to draw us inward, allowing us to have deep, restful sleep at night.

*Rajas,* or overactivity, is a constant companion in our modern world, encouraging us to literally or figuratively run in a hundred different directions and to experience as many of the infinite choices as possible. Primarily felt in the daytime hours, *Rajas* reaches its zenith at noon. All activity, including eating and digesting, is best accomplished when *Rajas* is supreme. The positive aspect of *Rajas* is that by trying many things and exploring many possibilities, we are sure to defeat the stasis of *Tamas*. The energy is now moving (if not in the most efficient way) and eventually a decision will be made, either by choice or through default.

*Sattwa* is when balance reigns. This could also be described as "dynamic stillness," a state in which motion and rest occur in perfect harmony.

During the interplay of *Tamas* and *Rajas,* one often becomes dominant while the other submits. Each comfortably rules its own domain.

Following the natural flow of the *gunas,* we live in balance. We are hindered when the *Rajas* and *Tamas* within us clash with the gentle flow of nature. Insomnia is a great example of this. The night, ruled by *Tamas,* is a time to go inward and rest. If at bedtime the mind is still racing in a *Rajasic* state, sleeplessness occurs. The busy mind, fed by *Rajas,* cannot surrender its activity to the needs of the body in *Tamas.* The body is then drawn into the *Rajasic* state as well, becoming restless and losing its much-needed time to cocoon. Allowing the mind to calm with quiet activities a few hours before bedtime, we more readily surrender to a great night's sleep, the ultimate *Tamas.*

When we overextend our energies during *Rajas* and fail to honor the indrawn time of night, *Tamas* will creep into our daylight hours. We may find ourselves tired or unable to think clearly, wanting to curl up and take a nap. Cloudy days that obscure the sun often invite *Tamas* to visit us.

At all times, to varying degrees, nature contains all three *gunas.* Ideally, we would like our temperament to settle into the quality of *Sattwa* all the time, but usually there is a great deal of fluctuation. There are times we may need to go well out of our way to invite *Sattwic* qualities back into our life. Once the invitation is accepted, the world becomes a harmonious venue for both action and inaction.

> One is elevated in consciousness when one experiences action in inaction, and inaction in action.
>
> —Bhagavad Gita

*When consciousness unites, it remains clear and unaffected by the external changes of nature, the gunas. This is the ultimate Vairagya.*

With continual Yoga practice, the body, mind, and emotions are able to narrow the ranges of both *Tamas* and *Rajas*. With this limiting, *Sattwa* is revealed and the deeper practices begin to divulge their transformational effect.

## THE MIND AND EMOTIONS AND THE MOON

To further help us understand this concept, imagine the moon and its cycles. From earth, the moon appears at certain times of the month to be half light and half dark. (It is actually difficult to see the half-dark portion, so it seems to be only half of the moon.) That is the time of *Sattwa,* a balance between dark and light. Within a few days the light increases until it fully illuminates the moon, and *Rajas* is present. With this full light of the moon, the mind and emotions are most active. Anyone who works at a hospital can attest to the chaos of a full moon. The patients are more restless and the emergency room is much fuller. Darkness then begins to obscure the light as the new moon, *Tamas,* begins to hold sway. With the dark or new moon, the mind and emotions are more indrawn; in extreme cases we may feel moody or even depressed.

*Tamas* often masquerades as *Sattwa.* Did you ever mistake your lack of ambition, or even a bit of depression, for a feeling of stillness and contentment? Perhaps you were able to fool others, but deep inside you knew you couldn't be further from tranquility. *Tamas* tends toward a lack of energetic consciousness, while *Sattwa* is an efficient and steady energy. When abiding in the *Tamasic guna,* we must transit through *Rajas* to embrace *Sattwa.*

If you're feeling lazy, a friend might encourage you to get up and *do something,* anything, to move the energy. Often hesitant to act because we are unwilling to make mistakes, we become immobilized (*Tamas*). By calling on *Rajas,* we may make many wrong turns, but at least we are moving. If after spinning our wheels we are able to spend a moment in stillness, we may discover that, miraculously, our center is rediscovered, and *Sattwa* is again with us.

With the glorious vision of the Self, nature's constantly changing temperament is unveiled. Through remembering, we honor the unchanging divinity in its eternal dance with our constantly changing humanity.

> If you become whole, everything will come to you.
>
> —*Tao Te Ching*

**When consciousness unites, it remains clear and unaffected by the external changes of nature, the gunas. This is the ultimate Vairagya.**

---

### EXPERIENCING THE EFFECT OF THE *GUNAS* (ATTRIBUTES OF NATURE) ON THE MIND AND EMOTIONS

*Notice your mind and feelings throughout the day. Sometimes you may feel yourself turning inward, while at other times you are active and energetic.*

*Do you feel in harmony with the dominant guna of the hour? Is that guna supporting you in what you need to do at that time?*

*When you feel out of balance, identify which guna you are in.*

*Be still for a few minutes and imagine that you are coming into balance.*

*If you are feeling Tamasic, do something active with your body, mind, or both.*

*If you are a bit Rajasic, do something to soothe yourself, like listening to quiet music or simply taking a few deep breaths.*

*Resist the temptation to feed the guna you are in. Ultimately, you will find a proven pathway to Sattwa as you discover ways to bring balance into your life.*

1.17 *By cultivation of Abhyasa and Vairagya, the intellect becomes keen, reasoning is clear, bliss is reflected to all, and outward identification unites with the Supreme Consciousness.*

1.18 *With continued awareness, we identify only with the pure consciousness residing in the heart.*

1.19 *Through identification with pure consciousness, the physical world can be transcended.*

1.20 *This identification is enhanced by faith, dynamism, intention, reflection, and perception.*

1.21 *To the dedicated and devoted, the divine truth is revealed.*

1.22 *Spiritual consciousness develops in direct proportion to one's dedication.*

CHAPTER

5

# BHAKTI YOGA:
## *Cultivating the Yoga of Devotion*

*B*HAKTI YOGA, or the Yoga of Devotion, is one of the most accessible and enjoyable ways to merge with the infinite. For many of us this way of devotion is omnipresent and seamlessly meshes with our own temperament.

*Boundless love and devotion unite us with the Divine Consciousness.*

*The Divine Consciousness is self-effulgent like the sun.*

*The Divine is the essence of all knowledge, wisdom, and love.*

*Knowledge, wisdom, and love are the omnipresent teachers, in all beings.*

*Repeating the sacred sound manifests Divine Consciousness.*

*When expressed with great devotion, the sacred sound reveals our divine nature.*

*By faithful repetition, the inner light luminously shines.*

# I.23 *Boundless love and devotion unite us with the Divine Consciousness.*

The secret to unleashing the power of devotion is now offered to us as *Bhakti Yoga.* Merging with the Divine through supreme devotion, *Iswara Pranidhana,* is such an important concept that we will see it repeated many more times in the Yoga Sutras.

## THE EVER-BLOSSOMING WAY OF *BHAKTI*

*Bhakti Yoga,* often seen as a mysterious path of devotion, is offered by the Yoga Sutras in a systematic form. In fact, its message is simple, and it seems almost strange that something as natural as opening our hearts has to be taught. After all, we arrive in this world with an open heart. But if it is not nurtured, that openness diminishes and is often unable to live past the limited duration of childhood. The sutras encourage us to continually cultivate that precious gift.

*Bhakti Yoga* in its various forms is the most widely embraced practice in the world. Also, *Bhakti,* not *Hatha,* is the most practiced form of Yoga! This may be because everyone, from the simple to the clever, can discover secrets of the heart.

*Bhakti* is often erroneously considered a path only for those possessing a highly emotional temperament. Images of weeping or chanting in rapture before an altar of the Divine are often associated with it. This is *one* aspect of *Bhakti* devotion, but be careful not to confuse *devotion* with *emotion.* True devotion and love shine through the Divine in every being.

Most of us traversing our particular way of devotion acknowledge that there is something beyond the individual "I." With an experience of great power, like standing on the shore of the boundless sea or witnessing the birth of a baby, we are embraced by feelings of gratitude *and* humility. These experiences link us to our hearts.

Like tomorrow's beautiful flower encased in a delicate bud, the expanded heart is, for many of us, still in a latent form. The heart, like the bud, protects itself from the harshness of the external world by staying cocooned, locking the Divine within. But through the continuous nurturing of deep devotion, the bud, in guarded increments, can expand its petals to fully blossom in all its beauty.

> To love means never to be afraid of the windstorms of life;
> should you shield the canyons from the windstorms you would
> never see the beauty of the carvings.
> —Elisabeth Kübler-Ross

*Boundless love and devotion unite us with the Divine Consciousness.*

## LEARNING TO LOVE LOVE

Unlike many of the practices, which tend toward precise instructions, there is no right or wrong way to love. Each one of us, in our own way, can express our wholehearted love of the Divine and of creation. Often as we tread lightly on this glorious path, the heart embraces the Divine in external form. It is always interesting for me to speak to individuals of the same faith about their personal relationship with the Divine, and to notice how differently each experiences it—as mother, father, friend, or something else entirely. Some identify the Divine with a name and a form, yet for others it is nameless and formless. Many imagine cosmic consciousness somewhere far away in heaven; for others it takes on a more accessible human form.

Often the Divine speaks through a person or a holy book. Within the same holy book, the Divine is described as wrathful, and loving, and spiteful, and compassionate. Which one is accurate? Could it be that we are projecting our own human traits and personalities onto the Divine? Could the Divine embody all of these qualities? Choose carefully which aspect you want to embrace, for "as you think, so you become." Whatever way you decide to show your devotion, *Bhakti* is one of the most natural ways for us to locate the ever-present Divine.

From our outward devotion we discover that the Divine *also* dwells within. At first it may appear as a small part of us, usually through some altruistic act. On performing an act of kindness, we may give credit to that glimmer of the indwelling Divine. "It is not me," we say, gesturing toward the sky. What happens when we are blamed? Hanging our heads, we refer to the dominant "human" perception of who we are and proclaim, "It's all my fault. I am not good enough."

Eventually, and perhaps after much discomfort, we arrive at the next stage of spiritual evolution, recognizing that, in good deeds and in bad, we are one with the Divine. The greatest challenge awaits us: to accept that the same Divine dwells in everyone!

## A WOMAN'S HEART

Honored by most traditions, a compassionate heart has become the symbol for devotion. It is often a female heart that is used as the standard for that devotion and love. In even the youngest of girls, care and nurturing for even the smallest creatures are intuitive and natural.

Motherhood has been anointed the apex of this love and compassion. Madonna and child was a familiar theme in the Christian church, even during times when wrathful images of the Divine were common. Worshippers longed for a compassionate image to speak to their hearts, and to intercede with the angry father. In such times, the mother often soothes the child and the father as well. Cultivate loving devotion, and you may find that it transforms everyone around you.


## A WOMAN'S TWO HEARTS

Women are graced with what is often referred to as the "womb heart." It relates to the "beating heart" through intuition and feelings. This legacy of love is so powerful that it is able to sustain a new life. The beating heart and womb heart each hold the sacred essence of consciousness. The capacity of our "beating" heart expands greatly as we experience infinite love; the overflow feeds us and others. To my joy, I found one ancient attempt in the Old Testament of the Bible to express the Divine as *Hiranya Garbha*, or the Golden Womb, the source of all beings that resides within each heart.

For many women, when the womb heart begins its metamorphosis to embrace a new life, the beating heart's capacity for love and devotion begins to expand. Our expectant mother now experiences three hearts within her: her beating heart, her womb heart, and the new soul's heart within her womb. Three pools of divine love. Is it any wonder we feel radiance emanating from an expectant mother? Everyone is drawn to her, with all three of her hearts active; she is directly sourcing divine love.

When it comes to love and devotion, motherhood holds the secret. Even those of us who have never physically given birth have within us the capacity and intuitive preparation for nurturing. All too often, in place of our heart's song, we listen to the intellectual values of our society cloaking our intuitive power. With grace, we can embrace both aspects, allowing the love and devotion to be channeled into the foundation of our lives.

*Boundless love and devotion unite us with the Divine*
*Consciousness.*

One of the most sincere ways devotion can be expressed is
through prayer. Try to find a time in your memory when you ab-
sentmindedly repeated a prayer in your chosen place of worship.
The words were being said, but they were probably being recited
by the mouth, not the heart. For prayer to reach its full power, the
heart must be the main speaker.

## A HUMBLE OFFERING OF GREAT DEVOTION

In the twilight of the predawn hours, after taking a ritual bath, simple women in India gather cow patties. Chanting prayers, hearts
overflowing with love and devotion, they roll the patties into sizable
balls. After infusing the Divine into these animal waste products,
they sweetly place a delicate flower on the crown of the mound.
The women then make offerings of water, rice, and flower petals to
further instill the Divine into the emerging form of Lord Ganesha,
the elephant god and the remover of obstacles.

To those of us growing up in a Western society, this seems like
a bizarre and unsanitary practice. If we look at it from this perspective, though, we miss the transformational aspect of simple
devotion.

Real love is possible only when you see everything as yourself.
—*Sri Swami Satchidananda*

When you drink the water, remember the spring from where it came.
—*Chinese proverb*

*Boundless love and devotion unite us with the Divine
Consciousness.*

## EXPERIENCING THE RHYTHM
## OF YOUR TWO HEARTS

*In a quiet room, sit or lie comfortably.*

*Choose a simple chant or prayer that touches your heart in a very
deep way.*

*Place one hand on your beating heart and the other on your
womb heart. (Even if your physical womb is not there, the energy
can still be summoned.)*

*With deep breaths, say the prayer aloud or silently, and begin to
feel the energy in each of the two hearts.*

*Notice if the energy of each has a different quality.*

*As the breathing and chanting continue, can you feel a balance
of energy between the two?*

*With the balance, experience the flow of love you feel for your
own child or loved one.*

*Then slowly continue to expand that love to others until it even-
tually embraces all.*

*Stay resting in that balance for as long as you like.*

*You can come to this practice anytime during the day when you discover you are missing that feeling of love. This allows you to embrace the Divine in everyday life.*

## 1.24 *The Divine Consciousness is self-effulgent like the sun.*

If the Divine is always in our hearts, then why would we need to do anything to call it forth? A contracted heart obscures the Divine within. With its opening, the Divine is revealed and we proclaim it as a miracle. The true miracle is that we are able to overcome doubt and experience that, with an open, loving heart, everything is possible.

**The Divine Consciousness is self-effulgent like the sun.**

## 1.25 *The Divine is the essence of all knowledge, wisdom, and love.*

## 1.26 *Knowledge, wisdom, and love are the omnipresent teachers, in all beings.*

In the ancient Yoga tradition, a spiritual teacher is called a *Sat Guru*, or teacher of truth. The word "guru" has two parts: "gu," that which hides our true light, and "ru," that which removes the covering. The word was traditionally reserved for a spiritual teacher of the highest regard; however, it has entered into common parlance and can even be found in the business pages of a newspaper.

Our mother is our first guru, teaching us the ways of love and of the world. Focused on her new treasure, she cares for us without judgment or expectations, and we are openly nourished by her infinite love. From the safety of our mother's heart, we are introduced to our father's wisdom. Later, our schoolteachers begin our study of the vast knowledge of the world. Eventually, the universe itself is revealed to us as our all-pervading teacher, a university of enormous proportions.

## IS A TEACHER ALWAYS A GURU?

In our lifetime we encounter any number of "teachers" who guide and educate us. For this ordinary accumulation of knowledge, there are many well-trained *uppa gurus* (worldly teachers) available to us. Most of us have had the privilege of being taught by a few inspiring teachers, while other teachers made us bolt at the sound of the school bell's ring.

Worldly teachers learn their knowledge from books and from their own teachers. They pass this information forward, usually discouraged from adding their own flavor to the teachings. Prospective teachers are often taught not to interpret, just to stick to the facts as they learned them. Often the teacher is not an expert in the subject but has a keen intellect that allows her or him to teach the subject so you can learn and refine your understanding.

These are fine attributes for an educator in the worldly sense, but not for a spiritual teacher. The spiritual guru must live what she or he teaches, as it is from truth that the power emanates.

Finding a true teacher in the uncharted territory of spirituality is challenging. Our relationship to the spiritual teacher requires enormous depth and commitment. We may be unable to grasp the vast scope of knowledge necessary to become awakened. Especially in these more skeptical times, the value of a living teacher is not appreciated. A true *Sat Guru* does not merely pass on her or his acquired knowledge; the guru also transmits Shakti (energy) from her or his vast reserves, to help kindle our own spark.

My guru, Swami Satchidanandaji, would often describe himself as yogurt culture. We, the students, were the hot milk, warmed by the fire of our practices. At the prescribed time the guru would transmit some of his Shakti energy to us by touching us on the top of the head, as if he were placing a little bit of live yogurt culture into milk. With that transmission of Shakti, our own energy began to grow and our devotion nurtured it. The culture continued to mature, transforming the milk into yogurt and moving our human consciousness closer to the Divine. In time, we are able to pass some of that culture to others. The guru initiates the student, who then becomes the guru and perpetuates the cycle. Yoga has for millennia been a tradition that directly transmits the power of its teachings from guru to disciple.

*The Divine is the essence of all knowledge, wisdom, and love.*

*Knowledge, wisdom, and love are the omnipresent teachers, in all beings.*

Choosing the right teacher is not always as easy as we would like. Place integrity at the top of the list when looking for a spiritual teacher. Many spiritual teachers reflect the teachings and their actions back to us through a mirror to show us who we truly are *and* the greatness that is our essential nature. Some show through their actions *exactly what we do not want to become.* Both are valuable. But much is also reported these days about gurus demanding that their students live an exemplary life, one that they themselves do not live. Before placing your total faith in a spiritual teacher, examine closely how she or he embodies the worldly *and* divine traits you wish to emulate.

Another important aspect is to always seek out a teacher who wants you to outshine her or him, not one who hopes to keep you in the student role forever. Learn as much from the guru on as many levels of your being as you are able. Let her or him be the link that will take you back to the essence of all teachings: the light within your own heart. When that spark is ignited, a true *Sat Guru* will be clear in letting you know that is not her or his light that she or he has given to you; instead, she or he has assisted you in rediscovering the same light of the Divine that shines in all. The purpose of seeking and learning from a guru is not to be bound but to be *free*. "When the student is ready, the guru appears." This well-known saying is often followed by a worthwhile addition: "When the student is ready, the guru disappears!"

## MAY THE GURU BE WITH YOU

It is not always necessary for the guru or teacher to be in physical proximity or even in the physical form to impart her or his Shakti. Many evolved souls guide us from other physical locations and realms. The subtle knows no boundaries. Spiritual support can come from the next town or from the far-reaching vistas we are yet to explore. For example, Lord Jesus, Lord Buddha, Lord Siva, Sri Krishna, Sri Radha, Sri Durga, Sri Lakshmi, Kwan Yin, Mother Mary, and others have successfully inspired devotees to find their divine essence for millennia. This is why the sutras say that the teacher of all teachers, the guru of gurus, is knowledge, wisdom, and love—boundless, eternal, pure, and unchanged by time.

Let your teacher be love itself.

—*Rumi*

*The Divine is the essence of all knowledge, wisdom, and love.*

*Knowledge, wisdom, and love are the omnipresent teachers, in all beings.*

## EXPERIENCING YOUR RELATIONSHIP TO THE INTERNAL OR EXTERNAL GURU

*Sit quietly and allow yourself to recall all the gurus and teachers who have taught you in the past and those who are guiding you now.*

*What lessons have you learned? How to act and how to be?*

*Were there some who showed you, by their words or actions, what not to do and how not to be?*

*Observing your present spiritual path, could a guru or a teacher enrich and increase the depth of your practice?*

*The first step in attracting a guru or a teacher is knowing that you are ready to receive guidance.*

*Set the intention and open your heart.*

*If you already have a guru or a teacher, are you able to accept the teachings wholeheartedly?*

*Does the guru or teacher live what she or he teaches?*

*Does she or he allow you to grow and flourish in your own personality?*

> *Recommit yourself to knowledge, wisdom, and love as the ulti-*
> *mate teachers.*

## I.27 *Repeating the sacred sound manifests Divine Consciousness.*

We are very much a verbal society—the word, it is said, is "might-ier than the sword." The old adage "Sticks and stones will break my bones but words will never hurt me" is patently untrue today. Lawsuits for saying hurtful words about someone are rampant. We can feel the power of words in the way they affect our emotions. A kind one can leave a smile on our face for hours; a cruel one can bring us to tears. This power of words can be seen in sacred texts as well.

The Rig Veda tells us, "In the beginning was *Brahman* [Divine Consciousness] as the sound and this sound truly was the supreme *Brahman*." This is almost identical to the Bible: "In the beginning was the word, and the word was with God and the word *was* God.". Often, when we visit an ancient place of worship, we can feel a special vibration. Sitting in a temple or a church causes our minds and hearts to be uplifted. This is the effect of many thousands of devoted prayers that reverberate in sacred vibration through the at-mosphere. Prayers in an ancient language radiate a special elevat-ing quality when repeated with a focused mind and an open heart. Even if you visit a holy shrine that is not of your tradition, you will likely find a sublime comfort there.

From the beginning of time there have been vibrations, or pulsa-tions, which eventually formed audible sounds. The sacred sound vibration is called a mantra. A mantra is name (*nama*), form (*rupa*), and action (karma) of Divine Consciousness. These mantras often do not have a literal meaning, but in our need to engage the intellect, we may assign them "meanings." A mantra is intended to transcend the mind by invoking a celestial sound, transporting us to a higher level of understanding.

"Mantra" has found its way into common usage. It is used to mean a word that, when spoken, wields its own power and transcends thoughts, emotions, and our ordinary view of the world.

*Repeating the sacred sound manifests Divine Consciousness.*

## REPEAT AS YOU LISTEN, LISTEN AS YOU REPEAT

The ancient prayers and sacred sounds from each tradition are calls, encouraging us to embark on our journey to the Divine. "Om," "amen," and "ameen" all hold the heartfelt feeling of the divine presence. Also, the peaceful vibrations of the Sanskrit "Om Shanti" mirror the Hebrew word for peace, "shalom." These vibrations seem to unite us, even when our traditions diverge.

*Love* is a wonderful vibration to choose. How adored you feel when someone says the words "I love you"! Love resonates in all languages throughout the world. Say "love" in French, *amour,* or Italian, *amore,* or Spanish, *amor.* Choose "love," or any phrase that, when repeated, reverberates within your entire being. Repeat it to yourself—one hundred, two hundred times a day.

This repetition of a sacred sound, word, or prayer is called *japa.* With each repetition, we become more in alignment with our true nature. When we hear it, see it, and say it, our bodies, minds, and worlds expand as the inner light is sparked.

## "OM": THE SACRED SOUND OF UNIVERSAL CONSCIOUSNESS

"Om" is the sacred mantra of divinity. It is chanted and revered as the sound from which all other sounds resonate, awakening universal consciousness. In this way it is the guru of sounds, invoking the Divine Consciousness in every sound.

The Mandukaya Upanishad expounds on the meaning of "Om," attempting to explain the simple essence of that sound. It divides "Om" into four sounds and stages. *A, U, M,* and the sound that is beyond all verbal pronunciation.

*A* is the beginning of all sounds. This is usually a baby's first sound, made simply by opening the mouth and saying "ah." The sound comes from the back of the tongue. Next the *U* sound, like "oo," is formed, moving forward in the mouth. And then, with the lips and teeth closed, the *M* is hummed.

*A-U-M* forms a trinity similar to other trinities that are more familiar: body, mind, spirit; creator, preserver, destroyer; past, present, future; the three *gunas;* Mother, Father, God; the Holy Trinity; and on and on. It brings all three prongs together in a simple sound.

Going beyond the trinity, the last bit of breath after the "Om" continues to be released without an audible sound to accompany it. This fourth part of "Om" is the unspoken sound, *Anahatha.* It is the vibration before and after all sound. If we listen closely after chanting, the resonance of the *mmm* sound can be felt, sometimes constant and sometimes oscillating. It is the sound of our merging with the infinite. This is the *Pranava,* the sound of *prana,* the divine energy.

All other Sanskrit mantras radiate from the root vibration "Om." Since "Om" is so subtle, other mantric vibrations are often added to allow the mantra to be more easily experienced. "Om Shanti" and "Om Namah Sivaya" are examples of this.

After a time of constant repetition, *japa,* the mantra will begin to repeat, seemingly by itself. At that time we enjoy listening. This listening is called *ajapa.* It is the sound of universal power rejuvenating itself.

With *japa,* the cells in our body and mind vibrate with that chosen sound as we assume the qualities. Today we have graphic machines that draw geometric patterns when certain sounds are produced. This concept existed centuries before in the yogic practice of repeating a mantra. When the sound "Om" and related mantras are chanted, a pattern is formed called a yantra (often called a mandala). Yogis saw and then reproduced these sacred drawings on paper and stone from their third eye. Even today the use of yantras as aids for focusing and meditation is honored.

> Truth is one. Many are the paths.
>
> *—Vedas*

*Repeating the sacred sound manifests Divine Consciousness.*

## EXPERIENCING "OM" AS DIVINE CONSCIOUSNESS BY REPEATING AND LISTENING

*Sit quietly and comfortably either on a chair or on the floor.*

*Align your head, neck, and spine. Expand your heart center.*

*Take in a few deep breaths to calm the body, mind, and emotions.*

*Begin to chant the sacred mantra "Om" in four distinct ways.*

*First, inhale deeply and pronounce the O longer than the M:*
OOOOOOOMMM.

*This enlivens the earth chakras (energy centers) and allows us a feeling of groundedness.*

*Repeat several times.*

*Second, inhale deeply and give the O and M sounds equal length:* OOOOOMMMMM.

*This brings balance to the earth and higher chakras.*

*Repeat several times.*

*Third, inhale deeply and elongate the M sound:* OOOMMMM.

*This brings awareness to the higher chakras for meditation.*

*Repeat several times.*

*Fourth, inhale deeply and chant "Om" with the elongated M as before. Then allow the breath to complete its exhalation without any audible sound, only listening:* OOOMMMMM . . . . . . . .

*This allows awareness to move to the highest levels of consciousness.*

*Repeat several times.*

*Be still and listen, and know that you are divine.*

## 1.28 *When expressed with great devotion, the sacred sound reveals our divine nature.*

The sacred sound must pluck the strings of our heart in order to unite our entire being. Often we are accustomed to repeating the same prayer, with our mind and heart engaged elsewhere. Then the prayer is only given lip service. The real grace comes when we are unified on all levels of our being.

*When expressed with great devotion, the sacred sound reveals our divine nature.*

## 1.29 *By faithful repetition, the inner light luminously shines.*

The real secret is to have a full and open heart when repeating a mantra or engaging in any spiritual practice. In the beginning, we are very concerned about correctly pronouncing the mantra or prayer. We may be "doing it exactly right," yet it may lack the most essential ingredient, devotion. The real power comes from the heart.

*By faithful repetition, the inner light luminously shines.*

### EXPERIENCING YOUR HEART'S SONG

*Sit comfortably in a chair or on the floor.*

*Choose a mantra or a prayer that allows your heart to fill with love. It does not matter if you do not know the meaning. The feeling is most important.*

*Begin to repeat this sacred sound aloud in a soft voice.*

*When, after some time, you are accustomed to the sound and feeling of the vibration, permit the lips and tongue to repeat the word delicately and thoughtfully, in a heartfelt whisper.*

*Moving further in, allow the heart to repeat it in silence. Feel the vibration moving in and out of your heart with each pulsation. Continue for a few minutes.*

*Allow the heart to overflow with the vibration and nourish your entire being. As you continue your day, the mantra will continue to repeat with each beat of your heart.*

*Feel that it is near and dear to you. Be faithful to it, and it will give you the secret to the power of the universe.*

# THE FOUR LOCKS AND FOUR KEYS:
## *Sustaining Equanimity*

These sutras speak about the potential imbalances we may encounter on the physical, mental, and emotional levels. They obscure the knowledge of our true nature. Offered are various ways to prevent these imbalances as well as ways to regain that precarious balance, if lost.

They show why the spiritual path is often likened to walking on a razor's edge.

*Perception of our true nature is often obscured by physical, mental, and emotional imbalances.*

*These imbalances can promote restlessness, uneven breathing, worry, and loss of hope.*

*These imbalances can be prevented from engaging by developing loyalty to a sacred practice.*

*To preserve openness of heart and calmness of mind, nurture these attitudes:*

*Kindness to those who are happy*

*Compassion for those who are less fortunate*

*Honor for those who embody noble qualities*

*Equanimity to those whose actions oppose your values*

*Slow, easeful exhalations can be used to restore and preserve balance.*

*Or engage the focus on an inspiring object.*

*Or cultivate devotion to the supreme, ever-blissful light within.*

*Or receive grace from a great soul who exudes divine qualities.*

*Or reflect on a peaceful feeling from an experience, a dream, or deep sleep.*

*Or dedicate yourself to anything that elevates and embraces your heart.*

I.30 *Perception of our true nature is often obscured by physical, mental, and emotional imbalances.*

I.31 *These imbalances can promote restlessness, uneven breathing, worry, and loss of hope.*

I.32 *These imbalances can be prevented from engaging by developing loyalty to a sacred practice.*

These sutras are understandable and do not seem to need further commentary. (They may be not as easy to put into practice as they are to comprehend!)

I.33 *To preserve openness of heart and calmness of mind, nurture these attitudes:*

> *Kindness to those who are happy*
> *Compassion for those who are less fortunate*
> *Honor for those who embody noble qualities*
> *Equanimity to those whose actions oppose your values*

This is a large dose of practical advice that allows us to integrate the highest spiritual values into our everyday lives. When we engage in the more "formal practices," that is, postures, breathing, or sitting in meditation, distractions often occur. We are affected by these distractions; however, they are more manageable when confined to our private world. Once we leave our sanctified space, the intrusions of the larger world present us with many more challenges.

Here we are offered four priceless keys that, if used in conjunction with the correct locks, open portals that enable us to retain our inner peace in all circumstances. The greatest challenge is to remember that *we hold the keys to our own peace.*

At first reading this sutra, we may think, "This is easy—of course I would react that way." As we begin to apply these subtle principles to our daily lives, we can trick ourselves into believing that we are kinder and more compassionate than we actually are. The ease manifests when thought, word, *and* deed mesh together.

These keys are also useful when reacting to our own actions, which can be even more complex than other people's actions. As the judging mind barges in, can the heart supersede it? Let's look at what a few of the challenges might be like. Of course, allow these to serve as examples that can help you explore the challenges in your own life.

### Kindness to those who are happy.

Imagine that you are meeting a friend whom you have not seen in ages. You pack a picnic and head to the park to catch up on what is happening in her life. Finding an ideal spot, you spread out a blanket, lay out the food, and begin to enjoy the tasty dishes and the wonderful company.

After the first two bites, both body and heart feel nourished. Just then a man sits down very close to you and lights up a big, fat, juicy cigar. Puffing happily, he leans back in the grass with a big grin, allowing the billowing smoke to waft directly into your nose and onto your food.

Before taking any action, observe your mind. Are you annoyed, even angry? "Who is *he* to ruin my perfect time by polluting us with cigar toxin!" Is judgment creeping in? Are you thinking how unconscious he must be to do something like that? "Is he doing it purposely to annoy me?"

Your blood pressure has probably risen, and your immune function is already weakened—not from the cigar toxin but from your own emotions and thoughts that have taken control.

Now give the heart a chance and look again at the man and the situation. He seems happy, relaxed, and at ease with the world, enjoying his treat. Do you want to spoil the mood and your own special time by responding to the situation with anger and self-righteousness? Those two emotions in particular can take hours to recover from.

Instead, try opening your heart and allowing kindness to meet his happiness. With a kind vibration, let the man know that you are happy he is enjoying his expensive cigar. Since you also would like to enjoy your meal, would he mind directing the smoke in another direction or, even better, enjoying it in another location? His response will often match the energy as well as the words you put forth.

Most situations in your life are not as dramatic, yet the same remedy will apply. Try overriding the mind's indignation with the heart's desire to love everyone. You may be amazed at the results.

*Compassion for those who are less fortunate.*

The word "compassion" is such a beautiful word; soft and gentle, it is composed of two parts: *com,* meaning "with," and *passion,* meaning "any intense emotion, either pleasurable or painful." Many times it is difficult to know which aspect of passion we are feeling, and sometimes we clearly encounter both at the same time.

Compassion is a form of infinite love, in that nothing can affect or limit it. It is extolled as a virtue for the very few, but is it? As women we seem to have a natural gift for radiating love and compassion. Our heartfelt compassion often embraces people in unfortunate circumstances beyond their control.

What, then, could prevail that would obscure this natural

quality? In certain circumstances a hesitation on our part may occur when someone is unhappy and needs our compassionate balm. Could our own worry and stress place compassion on the back burner?

Running late might be reason enough to create anxiety and prompt us to neglect our compassionate nature. If you feel rushed, a simple delay accelerates your anxiety. I think everyone has had this experience: You're waiting at a red light. Right as it changes to green, your foot comes off the brake, hovering above the gas pedal—you're ready to go! But traffic is not moving! Irritation mounts. You strain to look out the window, even give a toot on the horn. "Why are they not moving? The light is not going to get any greener! Probably someone's daydreaming or talking on her cellphone. I don't have all day! Let's go!" You're now in a fully adrenaline-charged state.

Imagine that when accelerating forcefully as the light turns from yellow to red, you notice out of the corner of your eye a blind woman and her guide dog safely finishing traversing the street. *That was the cause of the delay*—the very delay that caused you to be so irritated, anxious, and even angry. Observing the woman and her dog, your heart is again able to open and expand. The anger and annoyance dissipate, replaced by compassion.

The next time you are in a similar situation, recall this story and give the benefit of the doubt, allowing compassion to take over the driver's seat.

*Compassion for those who are less fortunate.*

Once we decide a person has a genuine reason for her suffering, our scope of compassion waxes and wanes according to how much we feel she "caused her own problem." Let's say that after getting fired from her third job, your friend comes to you for a compassionate ear. Each time she was fired, it was because she "borrowed" money from petty cash and was discovered. Your mind is thinking, "Well, she did it, *and* she got caught! She's smarter than that; why would she do such a thing? She doesn't need the money that much, does she?" Running wild with judgment and castigation, you plan your speech, based on "tough love." But she has already been reprimanded and suffered humiliation due to her actions. Out of work and defeated, she came to you seeking compassion and love. This is a perfect time to step back from the situation and reevaluate your role. Let your heart softly interrupt the blaming process and observe, "She seems so unhappy. Her heart is sad. She feels rejected and embarrassed and knows the next job will be harder to land because of her now very blemished record." Your part is to soothe her with a compassionate balm, rather than play a parental role and teach her a lesson. Whatever action people take, whether you approve of it or not, always make sure they know that you love them.

Through compassion you find that all human beings are just like you.

—His Holiness the Dalai Lama

*Compassion for those who are less fortunate.*

The way we treat others is often reflected in how we treat ourselves. When we are compassionate to those around us, it becomes easier to replicate that compassion when we are the one who caused a problem.

Did you ever press the wrong button on the computer and delete hours of work? Or perhaps you thought you set the oven to go on at a certain time but your dinner guests arrived to find dinner uncooked? At times like this, and in even more serious situations, having compassion for yourself is most important. Instead of calling yourself unkind names, take a moment to speak sweetly, as if to a child. "It's okay, sweetie, we can always call for takeout." This is when you need all the love and compassion you can soak up. For many of us, compassion is a one-way street going out of ourselves. Let it circle back around; use compassion as a soothing salve to treat everyone, starting with yourself!

> Compassion for myself is the most powerful healer of them all.
>
> —*Theodore Isaac Rubin*

### *Honor for those who embody noble qualities.*

Thanks to electronic news media, magazines, books, and the internet, historical information is in abundance, and most of us are fortunate to learn of great souls and their accomplishments. The opportunity for inspiration seems boundless. As we rejoice in and appreciate their qualities, we are inspired by knowing that such greatness is possible. If this dynamic feat can be done by one, why not by others? Much of what we need to achieve the extraordinary is encouragement and inspiration. The rest seems to take care of itself. Who are some of these great souls? We can probably agree on quite a few. Mother Teresa, Martin Luther King Jr., Mahatma Gandhi, Nelson Mandela, and others inspired miracles in our world. Through them and their deeds, the whole of humanity is elevated. There are also countless uncelebrated heroines and heroes among us, living their virtue quietly, whom we know little about.

Everyone has human limitations along with her or his greatness; it is up to us to choose which aspects to focus on. Observing noble qualities in others is a virtue of the heart. Our own horizons expand as we look toward the highest in others. Feeling discouraged, we may deflate our own talents while putting others on pedestals. "Oh, she is so talented; I could never dance like that." "She is such

a good cook. I always burn anything I bake." Or in our insecurity
we find reason to bring them down beneath us. "Yes, she might be
an extraordinary leader, but she is so wrapped up in her work that
she neglects her family."

Instead, try to find noble qualities in everyone. Some of us
may need to become archaeologists and dig deep. It could be as
simple as the graceful way she picks up a flower, or her keen fash-
ion sense, or his good work ethic. Whatever it is, no matter how
simple it may seem, focusing on this virtue will create a pathway
to our heart. The more we practice this way of relating to others,
the easier it is to recognize their divine qualities and ultimately
ours, too.

Spiritual teachers are everywhere, if our hearts are conditioned
to recognize them. These "ordinary people" have allowed me some
of my most precious learning experiences.

*Equanimity to those whose actions oppose your values.*

There are people and situations that make our blood pressure
spike by the mere mention of them. Certainly when we are offended by cruel or brutal acts, we feel we have the right to judge
and then seek retribution.

It would be a wonderful world if all people acted with honor and
consciousness. That, unfortunately, does not seem to be the way
of life in this age. We ourselves, at times, may have acted, spoken,
or thought unkindly, or hurt another person. Yet we are eager to
condemn, judge, and criticize others for doing so.

The Divine is present even in those who do unmentionable
atrocities. Granted, it is sometimes very hard to locate the Divine
in such people. Their minds and emotions are so disturbed and
clouded, it is difficult to perceive the goodness that resides within
them. For retaining *our* openness of heart and calmness of mind,
we must learn to forgive even the unforgivable.

The ultimate measure of a man is not where he stands
in moments of comfort and convenience,
but where he stands at times of challenge and controversy.
—*Dr. Martin Luther King Jr.*

The virtue of forgiveness is often misunderstood. There is a reluctance to grant it, for fear that it will let the offender "off the hook." But in truth, forgiveness is a natural stepping-stone to compassion. It gives us the opportunity to free others and ourselves. To hold hatred in our hearts is to clamp them tightly closed. Though the wrongdoer may feel the effects of our hate, we often suffer the most if we encase it within our hearts for too long. It erodes the very fiber of our love. It also binds us to the person we are condemning. By dwelling on the situation, we continually affirm that those who wronged us actually had the power to hurt us. This allows them to continue to hurt us! They become the object of our unkind focus. It is for our benefit, more so than for theirs, to see them as Divine Beings.

Forgiveness is a soothing balm vital to our health and happiness. If we grudgingly forgive, we still deem the other person responsible. "They did this to me, *but* I (in my generosity) will forgive them." As the heart softens through forgiveness, the understanding emerges that they are also hurt and unhappy, and then forgiveness melts into compassion.

Through compassion the identification of someone else as the perpetrator of our hurt vanishes. We understand that it is our perception that harms or heals. The same benevolent light shines within that person's heart as shines within ours.

*To preserve openness of heart and calmness of mind, nurture these attitudes:*

*Kindness to those who are happy*
*Compassion for those who are less fortunate*
*Honor for those who embody noble qualities*
*Equanimity to those whose actions oppose your values*

### EXPERIENCING USING THE RIGHT KEY TO UNLOCK THE ATTITUDE TO PRESERVE OPENNESS OF HEART AND CALMNESS OF MIND

*At the end of each day, take a few minutes to review the attitudes that you used freely.*

*Was there a situation where you applied the incorrect "key" and it did not unlock a feeling of peace?*

*Yet perhaps in another situation, the correct key opened an unexpected feeling of calmness.*

*In a journal, write down the lessons as you experienced them.*

*Reinforce the attitudes that you would like to incorporate into your life and alter the ones that no longer fit who you want to be.*

*Continue for several weeks and then appreciate how you have blossomed.*

1.34 *Slow, easeful exhalations can be used to restore and preserve balance.*

1.35 *Or engage the focus on an inspiring object.*

1.36 *Or cultivate devotion to the supreme, ever-blissful light within.*

1.37 *Or receive grace from a great soul who exudes divine qualities.*

1.38 *Or reflect on a peaceful feeling from an experience, a dream, or deep sleep.*

Retaining our balance and restoring it if lost are of utmost importance to our spiritual life. Recognizing that imbalance is the first step. Fortunately, once we know we are tipping that delicate balance, there are many ways to help restore our equilibrium. These sutras speak for themselves, giving us the guidance to regain our balance.

1.39 *Or dedicate yourself to anything that elevates and embraces your heart.*

Here we are given carte blanche to choose anything to which we want to dedicate our hearts. The preceding sutras have generously given us many wonderful suggestions for focusing the mind and the heart. Most people will find a suitable choice from within that group. If you do not find one that unlocks *your* heart, the sutras now invite you to create your own using two guiding principles.

First, choose something that will elevate you just by invoking its presence. And second, choose something that you love dearly and embrace it fully in your heart. If you are sincere and dedicated, you will be transported to its divine qualities and from there your inner peace will be unveiled. These are sure recipes for success in spiritual practice.

*Or dedicate yourself to anything that elevates and embraces your heart.*

# SAMADHI:
## *Merging with the Divine Consciousness*

FROM this sutra to the end of book I, we are introduced to the grand rewards of having focused our awareness on the highest, which then merges into varying states of union with our Divine Consciousness (*Samadhi*). The stages of *Samadhi* reflect the progressive withdrawal of individual consciousness (*chitta*) into the ocean of universal consciousness (*chit*). The various stages of the journey are presented in these sutras.

*Gradually through focused awareness one's knowledge extends from the smallest atom to the greatest magnitude.*

*As a naturally pure crystal appears to take the color of everything around it yet remains unchanged, the yogi's heart remains pure and unaffected by its surroundings while attaining a state of oneness with all. This is Samadhi.*

*When awareness merges with a "material" object or form, if the* name, quality, *and* knowledge *are perceived, this is* Savitarka Samadhi, *or reflective* Samadhi.

*When awareness merges with a "material" object or form, if* knowledge alone *is perceived, this is* Nirvitarka Samadhi, *or spontaneous* Samadhi.

*When awareness merges with a "subtle" object or form, two different* Samadhis *are present,* Savichara *(perceiving* name, quality, *and* knowledge*) and* Nirvichara *(perceiving* knowledge alone*).*

*These states of* Samadhi *have the power to extend beyond all the "material" and "subtle" forms and objects, to reveal nature in her unmanifested form.*

*All the* Samadhis *described thus far have been* Sabija *(with seed), which have the ability to germinate, returning us to ordinary consciousness.*

*In the purity of* Nirvichara Samadhi, *Divine Consciousness becomes luminescent.*

*When consciousness dwells in* absolute, true knowledge (Ritambhara Prajna), *direct spiritual perception dawns.*

*This* absolute, true knowledge (Ritambhara Prajna) *is totally different from the knowledge gained by personal experience, inference, and insights from the wise.*

*When experiencing this* absolute, true knowledge (Ritambhara Prajna), *all previous* Samskaras *(impressions) are left behind and new ones are prevented from sprouting.*

**Nirbija *(seedless)* Samadhi *outshines all impressions and manifestations.***

**1.40** *Gradually through focused awareness one's knowledge extends from the smallest atom to the greatest magnitude.*

Here we are inspired by the benefits that come from our diligent spiritual practice. Up to now the focused mind and emotions were directed toward an object or form. These practices allowed us to attain the spiritual power necessary for the next stage of elevating consciousness, *Samadhi*.

The hidden secrets of the universe may now be revealed to us. They could be the essence of the smallest atom or the most distant star. This does not occur through observation or theory. Rather, when we know ourselves, all other forms and objects are known to us. We understand that we are all one.

By knowing the one, we know everything.

—*Vedas*

*Gradually through focused awareness one's knowledge extends from the smallest atom to the greatest magnitude.*

**1.41** *As a naturally pure crystal appears to take the color of everything around it yet remains unchanged, the yogi's heart remains pure and unaffected by its surroundings while attaining a state of oneness with all. This is* Samadhi.

This realization is the fulfillment of the concept of *Vairagya* (remembrance of the Self) described in book I, sutra 15. When we hold fast to remembering we are the Divine Self, we merge with that Self. Even if the mind and emotions are temporarily distracted, the truth draws us back to the Self.

This sutra compares our consciousness to a perfectly clear crystal. When placed on a red cloth, it appears to be red. Once it is removed from the cloth, the flawless crystal is completely colorless again. We can repeat the action with a cloth of any color. Each time we can see that the color, which seemed to affect the crystal, in fact remains with the cloth. The crystal continues to reflect its true nature of purity and clarity.

Similarly, when we embrace the glory of knowing the Divine Self, our hearts and minds may appear to take on other characteristics. Yet as soon as we remember our True Self, there is immediate and complete recognition of the pure and unchanging Divine.

A great and mighty queen once gave an audience to a man whose immediate response was to ridicule the queen's way of governing the country. After a polite amount of time, she began to speak, interrupting his ranting.

"How would *you* react," she said with kindness, "if you brought me an enormous basket of the finest fruits and I said, 'No, thank you, I am not interested in keeping your gift.'" A bit startled, the man stammered, "It would distress me to think that you did not like my gift, but I would take back the basket of fruits and leave."

"Very well," said the queen calmly. "You have brought me a large basket of insults. Please take them away, as I do not wish to accept your offering."

In this story the queen took refuge in her true essence, remaining tranquil and secure even while the insults were attempting to cover her like a cloth. Each of us, like the queen, encounters people and things that try to coax us from the truth of knowing who we are. When we embrace this ever-present truth, we are free to live in joy within a constantly changing reality.

*As a naturally pure crystal appears to take the color of
everything around it yet remains unchanged, the yogi's heart
remains pure and unaffected by its surroundings while attaining
a state of oneness with all. This is* Samadhi.

### EXPERIENCING THE HEART AS A PURE CRYSTAL

*Sit quietly and, with focused awareness, imagine your heart as
a pure crystal.*

*Appreciate its clear, reflective quality.*

*Now begin to remember a situation or emotion. If possible, place
a color value on it. (If it made you angry, for instance, it might
reflect red.)*

*Slowly bring the situation or emotion reflected in the color near
the pure crystal of your heart.*

*Notice if the crystal is affected by the color. Is the heart affected
by the situation? Do your feelings release a color?*

*Observe if the mind and emotions engage and support the situa-
tion or the clarity of the heart crystal.*

*Now, with great care, remove the situation and the color from
the crystal's reflection.*

*Does the heart crystal hold any of the color, or has it stayed true
to its pure and reflective nature?*

*Use this frequently to remember your true divine nature.*

I.42 *When awareness merges with a "material"*
*object or form, if the* name, quality, *and* knowledge
*are perceived, this is* Savitarka Samadhi, *or reflective*
Samadhi.

Once we have ascended through *Dharana,* contemplation, and
*Dhyana,* meditation (book III, sutras 1–2), our awareness, inspired
by the various suggestions offered in the previous sutras, is able to
merge with the "material" object or form we have chosen. This is
*Savitarka,* the first stage of *Samadhi.*

In *Savitarka Samadhi,* the awareness no longer wanders from
the object itself (as it did in *Dharana* and *Dhyana*); instead it flut-
ters among the name of the object, its quality, and the knowledge
enveloped in the object.

In its simplest form, if we join our focused awareness to a candle
flame ("material" object), we have identified it by its *name,* "flame."
We recognize the *qualities* of light and heat. The *knowledge* of the
flame relates to our own observation that it gives light. After identifying all three attributes, our thoughts and feelings begin to wander, in an inconsistent pattern, to *name, quality,* and the *knowledge*
they hold. With each new visit to one aspect or another, new variations will emerge. This keeps the mind and emotions engaged in
movement.

Because the movements are slight, our focus is able to deepen
and we alight in *Savitarka Samadhi.* Reaching this stage is a grace
that is enhanced by a feeling of gratitude. The constant waver-
ing, although negligible, is enough to prevent us from attaining the
state of full transcendental awareness.

*When awareness merges with a "material" object or form, if the*
name, quality, *and* knowledge *are perceived, this is* Savitarka
Samadhi, *or* reflective Samadhi.

I.43 *When awareness merges with a "material"*
*object or form, if* knowledge alone *is perceived, this is*
Nirvitarka Samadhi, *or spontaneous* Samadhi.

In this stage of *Samadhi,* identification with the "material" form of
an object (its name and quality) retreats, and knowledge is all that
remains. The awareness no longer wanders but merges with the
essential perception of the "material" form or object.

Using the example of the candle flame, the identification with
the name "flame" or even the quality of light or heat is absent in
*Nirvitarka Samadhi.* Instead a higher knowledge beyond the senses
allows us to know the flame's unseen characteristics. We have acquired knowledge of the origin and purpose of its light.

Albert Einstein, the great scientist and visionary, was often asked
how he discovered the intimate properties of something as subtle
as light. It was not the laboratory testing that led to the discovery
as much as the many years spent contemplating and meditating on
the secrets concealed in light. When he ultimately merged with
light in *Nirvitarka Samadhi,* all its secrets were revealed.

With *Nirvitarka Samadhi* we boldly enter the realm of mystical
understanding, encountering a web of intricacies that are beyond
the grasp of the logical mind.

*When awareness merges with a "material" object or form, if*
knowledge alone *is perceived, this is* Nirvitarka Samadhi, *or*
*spontaneous* Samadhi.

## EXPERIENCING MERGING AWARENESS WITH A "MATERIAL" OBJECT OR FORM

(Please note: This practice is presented to help us to understand *Savitarka* and *Nirvitarka Samadhi*. It is not intended to induce the state itself. If it does occur, however, it is known as *grace*.)

*Sit comfortably with a lit candle at eye level.*

*Begin to repeat the name "flame" in silent repetition.*

*Feel the quality of heat and light that the flame emits.*

*Experience the secret knowledge of how light emanates from the flame.*

*Then go back over the three parts, allowing the thoughts and feelings to stay with the three attributes.*

*Notice when the awareness wanders, and gently refocus on the name, quality, and knowledge of the flame.*

*Let the name and quality fade and perceive only the essence of clear light.*

*As you return to material awareness, notice where your consciousness has led you.*

1.44 *When awareness merges with a "subtle" object or form, two different* Samadhis *are present,* Savichara *(perceiving* name, quality, *and* knowledge*) and* Nirvichara *(perceiving* knowledge alone*).*

These are both higher stages of *Samadhi* than those previously discussed. With both *Savitarka* and *Nirvitarka Samadhi,* we are obliged by language and our five senses to present the concept of a "material" object or form in order to access its knowledge.

With both *Savichara* and *Nirvichara Samadhi,* knowledge is gained through merging awareness with "subtle" forms and objects. In *Savichara Samadhi,* there is again a vacillation among *name, quality,* and *knowledge;* the three remain separate, without blending. In *Nirvichara Samadhi, name* and *quality* blend, releasing *knowledge* alone to merge with our awareness.

These *Samadhis* are more difficult to comprehend, as they are outside the ordinary confines of language and outside of time and space as we know it. Being subtler, they elicit a deeper focus to reveal their essence.

Some examples include meditating on a sacred mantra (especially in the ancient Sanskrit language); the chakras (energy vortexes), which hold thought, emotional patterns, and karmic forecasts; or one of the five subtle elements (*Tanmatras*) housed in the chakras. These "subtle" forms and objects may also include elevated thought or emotional forms, such as love, compassion, intuition, and so on.

For an example, the *Anahatha* chakra (heart chakra) is in the "subtle" rather than the "material" form and cannot be experienced through our five external senses. We are, however, able to merge awareness with the *Anahatha* chakra as a vessel emanating infinite love and compassion and experience that love and compassion in our lives. This is *Savichara Samadhi.*

When infinite love and compassion are experienced and nothing else fills the awareness, *Nirvichara Samadhi* is experienced.

This new level of consciousness is without cause or effect, place or time. The inexpressible states of pure bliss (*Sa-ananda Samadhi*) and the effulgence of the pure Self (*Sa-asmita Samadhi*) that follow *Nirvichara Samadhi* allow us to radiate infinite love and compassion to all.

*When awareness merges with a "subtle" object or form, two different* **Samadhis** *are present,* **Savichara** *(perceiving* name, quality, *and* knowledge) *and* **Nirvichara** *(perceiving* knowledge alone).

## EXPERIENCING MERGING AWARENESS WITH A "SUBTLE" OBJECT OR FORM

(Please note: This practice is to help us to understand *Savichara* and *Nirvichara Samadhi*. It is not intended to induce the state itself. If it does occur, however, it is known as *grace*.)

*Sit comfortably.*

*Begin to repeat the name "Anahatha chakra" silently.*

*Feel the quality of infinite love and compassion this chakra emanates from the center of your heart.*

*Allow the knowledge of how love and compassion emanate from the Anahatha chakra to come to you.*

*Allow the thoughts and feelings to merge awareness with the name, quality, and knowledge of the Anahatha chakra.*

*Let the name and quality fade and allow yourself to be bathed
in the knowledge of infinite love and compassion, the essence of
the Anahatha chakra.*

*As you return to material awareness, notice where your con-
sciousness has led you.*

## 1.45 *These states of Samadhi have the power to extend beyond all the "material" and "subtle" forms and objects, to reveal nature in her unmanifested form.*

Our awareness becomes focused first on the "material" and then
on the "subtle" elements. Their far-reaching power leads us to the
essence of manifested energy and then to nature in her unmanifested form (*Prakriti*). Here is where we meet the three *gunas* (attributes of nature), equal and in balance with one another.

With the slightest fluctuation, the delicate balance of energy is
reordered, resulting in the manifestation of all phenomenal matter
(creation). So even in these elevated stages of *Samadhi,* we are still
unable to merge completely with the True Self. In order for us to
directly unite with the Divine, we must traverse and then transcend the phenomenal worlds, both manifested and unmanifested.

*These states of Samadhi have the power to extend beyond all
the "material" and "subtle" forms and objects, to reveal nature
in her unmanifested form.*

**1.46** *All the* Samadhis *described thus far have been* Sabija *(with seed), which have the ability to germinate, returning us to ordinary consciousness.*

We have climbed the lofty stages of *Samadhi* only to learn of its impermanence. The term *Sabija* (with seed) reminds us that the bliss of this higher state is temporary, and our ordinary ways of thinking and feeling can reappear at any moment.

Although these *Samadhis* are of a higher order than most of our spiritual practices, they still have only a limited amount of power to sustain consciousness in that exalted state for an extended time. It can last for minutes or days, but at some point our awareness returns to individual consciousness. This is due to the fertile seeds holding our thoughts, emotions, and karmas. (Karma will be described in book II, sutras 12–14.) However, if we continue to steady the mind and heart, these states of *Samadhi* will become more frequent and a natural ascension will occur.

*All the* **Samadhis** *described thus far have been* **Sabija** *(with seed), which have the ability to germinate, returning us to ordinary consciousness.*

**1.47** *In the purity of* Nirvichara Samadhi, *Divine Consciousness becomes luminescent.*

In *Nirvichara Samadhi* (perceiving knowledge of subtle forms alone), the (karmic) seeds, while still present, are less likely to germinate. Having progressed this far, it is always possible to return to individual consciousness, but it is less likely because of the strong and continuous identification with the light of the Divine Self. Each time a greater part of our consciousness remembers these transcendental states and longs to reside in them, they become more intoxicating than our former awareness.

*In the purity of* **Nirvichara Samadhi,** *Divine Consciousness becomes luminescent.*

1.48 *When consciousness dwells in* absolute, true knowledge (Ritambhara Prajna), *direct spiritual perception dawns.*

1.49 *This* absolute, true knowledge (Ritambhara Prajna) *is totally different from the knowledge gained by personal experience, inference, and insights from the wise.*

1.50 *When experiencing this* absolute, true knowledge (Ritambhara Prajna), *all previous* Samskaras *(impressions) are left behind and new ones are prevented from sprouting.*

This absolute, true knowledge (*Ritambhara Prajna*) differs from the learned knowledge described in book I, sutra 6. The previous knowledge derived from books, spoken words, or the senses is no longer sufficient to satisfy the deep yearning for truth.

This higher absolute, true knowledge is directly imparted to us by an unseen grace. In previous stages of *Samadhi* there may have been the need for guidance from our minds or hearts (i.e., stay alert, center on the object, etc.) to help us focus and maintain awareness. At this level there is a magnetic power of attraction that effortlessly draws us toward the *Ritambhara Prajna*.

*When consciousness dwells in* absolute, true knowledge
(Ritambhara Prajna), *direct spiritual perception dawns.*

*This* absolute, true knowledge (Ritambhara Prajna) *is totally
different from the knowledge gained by personal experience,
inference, and insights from the wise.*

*When experiencing this* absolute, true knowledge (Ritambhara
Prajna), *all previous* Samskaras *(impressions) are left behind
and new ones are prevented from sprouting.*

## 1.51 Nirbija *(seedless)* Samadhi *outshines all impressions and manifestations.*

In this highest stage of *Samadhi,* the immortal Divine Self shines.
All the other seeds and *Samskaras* (past impressions) have been
rendered impotent. With all the *Sabija* (with seed) *Samadhis,* there
is still a kernel of the subtle awareness of "I." With *Nirbija* (seedless) *Samadhi,* the illusions of birth and death have fled, and in
their place is simply the knowledge of the immortal Divine Self.

   Living in the world in this *Samadhi,* we emanate total compassion and love, and our hearts and minds are forever united with
the one Divine Consciousness that we perceive in all. This is the
ultimate *Samadhi,* complete and everlasting union with the Divine.

> Pilgrim, pilgrimage, and road—it was but myself toward my Self,
> and your arrival was but myself at my own door.
>
> —*Rumi*

*Nirbija* (seedless) *Samadhi outshines all impressions and
manifestations.*

(Please note: It is my experience that while these states of *Samadhi* are interesting to know about and can enlighten us as to the great heights we may reach, they can also veer us away from the practical. They are not states that we can *attain;* instead they are the fulfillment of our conscious evolution. My assurance to you is that, as your consciousness traverses these levels, the names and their meanings will be useless. If even for a moment your mind searches for the names or attributes of each of the *Samadhis,* you will again be back to the world of thoughts and feelings. Instead, as you visit or make a permanent residence in these exalted stages of *Samadhi,* enjoy the experience.

BOOK II

# SADHANA PADA

*Cultivation of Spiritual Practice*

Book II, "Sadhana Pada: *Cultivation of Spiritual Practice*,"
reveals the practices and experiences that encourage the reunion of
consciousness.

When we venture inward, it is useful to have a guide or even a road
map. Sadhana Pada lays out a splendid array of practices that can
appeal to anyone at any stage. The practices are presented twofold:
in bite-sized pieces ready to be embedded in your daily life and as the
more formal practices that require stillness.

# KRIYA YOGA:
## *The Venerable Threefold Path*

K RIYA YOGA embraces the venerable threefold path of: *Karma Yoga,* dedicated service to all; *Jnana Yoga,* intuitive wisdom; and *Bhakti Yoga,* love and devotion.

*Kriya Yoga,* or Yoga in action, embraces:

*Tapas:* igniting the purifying flame

*Swadhaya:* sacred study of the Divine through scripture, nature, and introspection

*Iswara Pranidhana:* wholehearted dedication to the Divine Light in all

*These practices enhance inner awareness and guide us to liberation.*

## II.I Kriya Yoga, *or Yoga in action, embraces:*

*Tapas:* igniting the purifying flame

*Swadhaya:* sacred study of the
Divine through scripture, nature, and introspection

*Iswara Pranidhana:* wholehearted dedication to the Divine
Light in all

## II.2 *These practices enhance inner awareness and guide us to liberation.*

*Kriya Yoga,* or Yoga in action, seamlessly weaves the teachings of Yoga into our everyday world, becoming a template for our hands, heads, and hearts to follow. When mixed in the correct proportions, action, thought, and feelings harmonize completely, allowing our inner spirit and the outer world to unite.

The practice of *Tapas* reflects *Karma Yoga* (dedicated service to all) and invites us to embrace all experiences without expecting any specific results. With this attitude, the purifying flame is ignited. The material world graciously stands ready with multiple opportunities for self-improvement and purification. The true reward is to understand and accept all challenges as gifts that enhance clarity.

*Swadhaya* reflects *Jnana Yoga,* encouraging us to consider and study the divine and natural realms and to examine ourselves just as carefully. Fine-tuning our mental and intuitive aspects, we harmonize with the inspirations that they have to offer.

*Iswara Pranidhana* is an aspect of *Bhakti Yoga,* the recently discussed practice of wholehearted dedication to the Divine Light in all. Through this practice, the intoxication of the Divine is made present at every moment and with every action.

> The hand stays in society while the heart rests with the Divine.
> —Bhagavad Gita

This is a mighty and blessed formula.

## THE GODDESS GAYATRI BREATHES LIFE INTO THE WORLD

The same triad of power present in *Kriya Yoga* is reflected most simply in the ancient Gayatri mantra. This sacred mantra is the universal prayer enshrined in the Rig Veda. Chanted for thousands of years, it invokes the Divine Light, honored through the ages as the source of our continued creation. By dedicated repetition of Gayatri, all the wisdom and practices of *Kriya Yoga* can be experienced.

The sacred prayer is dedicated to the goddess Gayatri, a feminine aspect of pure consciousness who is considered to be the mother of the Vedas. From Divine Light she creates all life. She resides within the heart of human souls as she outwardly enhances the splendor of the natural world.

Until recently this mantra was kept in strict secrecy. Only those purified by initiation were permitted to hear this sacred prayer, let alone chant it, as they yearned for its dynamic power of liberation. The goddess Gayatri in her compassion has recently offered this transformational mantra to the uninitiated secular world. Its powerful and purifying effects permeate all environments, affecting the entire globe on profound levels. Chanting along to a recording of the Gayatri mantra, or even just listening to it, one readily experiences its power.

The sacred Gayatri mantra is a unique way to understand *Kriya Yoga*. It deepens spiritual understanding without the intervention of the mind. Repetition of the mantra channels its vibratory meaning directly to the heart.

> *Om Bhur Bhuvah Swaha*
> *Tat Savitur Varenyam*
> *Bhargo Devasya Dhimahi*
> *Dhiyo Yonah Prachodayat*

> Embracing earth, heaven and beyond
> The sacred source is revealed
> Evoking the resplendent flame
> The all-pervading light venerates us all.

**Kriya Yoga,** *or Yoga in action, embraces*
   **Swadhaya:** *sacred study of the Divine through scripture, nature, and introspection*

> *From Gayatri*
> *Om Bhur Bhuvah Swaha / Tat Savitur Varenyam*
> **Embracing earth, heaven, and beyond / the sacred source is revealed**

The first two lines of the Gayatri mantra represent reflective study on all three levels encased in the Divine and natural realms, and this relates to *Swadhaya*. *Bhur* refers to the earth, *Bhuvah* the heavens, and *Swaha* the higher consciousness beyond the worlds we know (notice that "swa" is also the first part of *Swadhaya*). With study we are able to ascend to the highest level, to the source we hold sacred.

## TO STUDY IS TO LOVE

*Swadhaya* study comes in many forms. To aid in our worldly and divine studies, we are blessed to have an extensive range of books available to us. With that availability comes the responsibility to cultivate a high level of discrimination. Adapting study as a spiritual practice addresses our social responsibility as well as that of our intellect.

As Paramahansa Yogananda once said, "Read a sentence from a book and when you have incorporated it into your life go on to the next sentence." This great quote gives us a glimpse into the quality of study we are seeking as well as the devotion and dedication necessary. Evaluate the books you are reading. Are your books stimulating your consciousness, inspiring you to do great things? Or are they just inspiring dust to collect? Better to have a few choice books that encourage you than a huge library that clutters your shelves and your mind. Books can be great teachers when they encourage us to take the high road and bestow compassion on others. Many people still read and adhere to the time-honored classics because, in one form or another, they pass on this gem of wisdom.

*Swadhaya* also encourages study of the natural world by observing with awe her bounty and the uniqueness of everyday life. Greet the morning light with reverence and wonder, and with the diminishing light welcome the miracle of night as you draw inward. Let each butterfly and ant have a delightful presence in your life. Study nature and feel the comfort of her presence.

Children are our best teachers for studying nature. Ever take a walk with a three- or four-year-old? You might have said something like "Come on, honey, we can't stop and look at every little bug!" Instead of teaching our children to hurry, let the babes teach us to marvel at nature.

Kriya Yoga, *or Yoga in action, embraces*
   Swadhaya: *sacred study of the Divine through scripture,
   nature, and introspection*

   *From Gayatri*
      *Om Bhur Bhuvah Swaha / Tat Savitur Varenyam*
      **Embracing earth, heaven, and beyond / The sacred
         source is revealed**

When we embark on a journey of introspection or a deep study
of ourselves, we tend to see the surface of our bodies and recognize
the shortcomings. Perhaps we notice a few more wrinkles, another
gray hair, that chocolate éclair that went straight to the hips. How
different we would feel if we took the time to really look at the
miracle of life and repeat a gentle phrase or affirmation, a smile
of recognition. Remind yourself constantly that you are a Divine
Being, nothing more, nothing less, and nothing else! To know and
love the higher aspect of yourself is an exquisite way to practice
*Swadhaya.*

## THE SEED OF THE UNIVERSE

Within the aspect of *Swadhaya* are prayer and *japa* (repetition of
a mantra).
   A mantra is a one- or many-syllable sound that transcends the
mind and emotions. If repeated for its vibrational effect, it brings
us to the level of *Swaha.* A mantra is like a seed: Its simplicity
hides the potential power it holds. Seeing a tiny acorn, it is difficult to imagine the mighty oak tree within. Likewise, though
it might not seem like much, the smallest mantra (like "Om"),
when repeated with the heart, has the power to unite us with our
divine nature.

Swadhaya: *sacred study of the Divine through scripture, nature, and introspection*

> Om Bhur Bhuvah Swaha / Tat Savitur Varenyam
> *Embracing earth, heaven, and beyond / The sacred source is revealed*

Kriya Yoga, *or Yoga in action, embraces*
  Tapas: *igniting the purifying flame*

> *From Gayatri*
> *Bhargo Devasya Dhimahi . . .*
> *Evoking the resplendent flame*

*Tapas* is taken literally to mean "burn" or "purify." In a higher sense it is an attitude that allows us to embrace all of life's experiences as a means for purification, be they pleasant or unpleasant.

A truckload of gold ore would appear to most of us as a bunch of ordinary black rocks. To be purified, the ore is heaved into a scalding hot fire. The impurities slowly turn to ash, leaving a minute quantity of sparkling purified gold (alchemy at play). Gold's worth is measured by its purity, so the longer it remains in the fire, the more refined—and more valuable—it becomes. First it becomes twelve karats, then fourteen, and with continued firing, the purest and most precious twenty-four-karat gold emerges.

For most traditions this kind of refinement is made available to our consciousness through *Karma Yoga*, the path of selfless service, the alchemy that purifies the heart and mind. Often in the name of spiritual growth, *Tapas* will be interpreted as asceticism. This is an unfortunate euphemism for overworking or even harming the body, mind, and emotions. In an effort to "detach" from the "pleasures" of the body, people are known to fast for prolonged periods of time, stand on one leg for days, lie on beds of nails, walk on hot coals, wear hair shirts, and partake in any number of practices to induce pain. They think that anything that magnifies discomfort will surely burn away impurities and control the mind! Often, though, the opposite occurs as the body and mind cry out for comfort and relief. Many of these austerities can also seriously damage the body, defacing the temple that houses the divine spirit.

> Those who seek to destroy the body also destroy me, the indweller.
> —Bhagavad Gita

Although outwardly very spectacular, these austerities are *not* the highest form of *Tapas*. Conjuring up any form of *Tapas* is not really necessary, as it seems that with each new day the world serves up new challenges by which we are purified. If we intentionally add discomfort or pain to an already weakened body or mind, this tends to further separate us from the divine spirit. Pay close attention in your own life to how *Tapas* manifests. Its hardships may even persuade you to doubt the existence of the Divine—but in the end, see if you aren't purified by its flames.

**Kriya Yoga,** *or Yoga in action, embraces*
  **Tapas:** *igniting the purifying flame*

> *From Gayatri*
>   *Bhargo Devasya Dhimahi . . .*
>   *Evoking the resplendent flame*

## THE OPPORTUNITIES FOR *TAPAS* ARE UNLIMITED

Imagine you have been driving around looking for parking and, just as you are backing into a space, someone barges in and takes it.

Or maybe you are on the freeway and a car cuts in front of you, causing you to brake quickly. Can you avoid shifting that anger and frustration onto yourself or those around you? Are you able to embrace these emotions and inconveniences as a means for purification, or do they give you a good excuse to curse and shout?

What if it is not a human disturbance but an external one, like a dead car battery? The car is already packed; you are ready to embark on a much-needed weekend away. Your route is mapped out to miss the stream of traffic on Friday night. You turn the ignition and nothing happens! The hope of missing the traffic and getting to your destination before dark is completely lost. Do you see it as a wonderful time to manage the frustration you are holding in the mind and emotions, or is it an excuse to scream at the next person who detains you? How we react to these situations becomes the framework of our spiritual practice.

Even the most minute of disturbances during our formal Yoga practices can send us plummeting from the higher realms back to the material world. A tiny mosquito buzzing in your ear during deep relaxation can quickly turn the practice into an arm-waving event worthy of Olympic competition. If, though, we use *Tapas* to tether ourselves close to our center, its transcendent power moves with us into daily life.

The more luminescent we are, the more we are able to serve without wanting rewards. If an unpleasant situation should occur, we accept it as a means for purification, returning only joy and love. This is considered one of the best and most challenging forms of *Tapas*. The supreme purpose of *Tapas* is to accept life's challenges while being loving and compassionate to all, especially ourselves.

At times it might feel as if we are doled a greater portion of *Tapas* than we can handle. Those are the times to draw upon the strength we have gained from the formal practices, and to be grateful for it (if we can).

Mother Teresa of Calcutta was asked during a moment of great trial if she thought Jesus ever tested her beyond her limits. She hesitated slightly before she responded: "No, I don't think I am ever tested beyond my limits, but I often wish He did not have such a high opinion of me!"

**Kriya Yoga,** *or Yoga in action, embraces*
  Tapas: *igniting the purifying flame*

> *From Gayatri*
>   *Bhargo Devasya Dhimahi . . .*
>   ***Evoking the resplendent flame***

**Kriya Yoga,** *or Yoga in action, embraces*
  Iswara Pranidhana: ***wholehearted dedication to the Divine Light in all***

> *From Gayatri*
>   *Dhiyo Yonah Prachodayat*
>   ***The all-pervading light venerates us all***

*Iswara Pranidhana* is a recurrent theme throughout the sutras. It is often considered one of the most pleasing and among the easiest of practices.

By sprinkling life with devotion, we can transform each and every moment of it. Our ultimate awakening may come simply by pausing regularly to feel this wholehearted dedication to the all-pervading light within.

The human mind has difficulty comprehending something as vast as an all-pervading omniscient consciousness. Throughout its history, human society has narcissistically associated its own image with that of the Divine. Further evolution of this concept projected a human *male* likeness onto the formless, solidifying the exclusivity of male divinity. The writers and translators, almost exclusively men themselves, endorsed this characterization. Up until very recently, the masculine nature of the Divine was an undisputed reality.

As women, our experience of the divine energy is often found in communion with the changing cycles of nature, in the joys we reap from our personal relationships, in the love of our families. Our dedication and devotion, while easily expressed, are often un-reciprocated. Frequently, in the search for returned affection, we lavish our wholehearted devotion on one or more masculine images (fathers, sons, husbands, ministers, priests, rabbis, teachers, etc.), ignoring the Divine within ourselves. We need to discover ways to value our own power even as our hearts remain entwined with others.

By delving into our hearts, we pass the boundaries of our lim-ited minds and recognize the Divine Consciousness as primordial energy within each living thing. A person, an animal, a falling leaf, or a sinking stone—all are part of the Divine. When we make this realization with our hearts, we are drawn in love to the divine en-ergy in all things, and the whole world becomes our beloved. How could it really be otherwise?

Kriya Yoga, *or Yoga in action, embraces:*
Iswara Pranidhana: *wholehearted dedication to the Divine Light in all*

*From Gayatri*
*Dhiyo Yonah Prachodayat*
**The all-pervading light venerates us all**

## EXPERIENCING *KRIYA YOGA* THROUGH
## CHANTING OF THE GAYATRI MANTRA

*Learn and begin to repeat the Gayatri mantra a few times a day.*

*As you hear the Sanskrit, remind yourself of the translation in English. Understand and experience the words as their truth resonates in your heart.*

> *Om Bhur Bhuvah Swaha Tat*
> *Savitur Varenyam Bhargo*
> *Devasya Dhimahi Dhiyo*
> *Yonah Prachodayat*

Embracing earth, heaven, and beyond
The sacred source is revealed [reflecting *Swadhaya*]
Evoking the resplendent flame [reflecting *Tapas*]
The all-pervading light venerates us all [reflecting *Iswara Pranidhana*]

*After a time, let go of the literal meaning and just focus on the vibration. Notice how it resonates in your heart, reverberating through your body, thoughts, and emotions, glazing your entire life. (If this is an unfamiliar chant, you can listen to one of the many recordings available on the internet. Find one with a tune that resonates with your heart and is easy to chant along with.)*

*After the formal sitting, enjoy the Gayatri mantra playing in the background while you work or play. The meaning will continue to vibrate within your heart.*

## EXPERIENCING *KRIYA YOGA* IN EVERYDAY LIFE

*Observe the different aspects of* Kriya Yoga *and how you've prac-*
*ticed them throughout the day.*

*Create a practice for each of the three aspects of* Kriya Yoga
*that is meaningful to you. Change or alter the practices as you*
*choose.*

*What would your practice of* Karma Yoga *(selfless service) and*
Tapas *(igniting the purifying flame) be like?*

*What would your practice of* Jnana Yoga *(Intuitive Wisdom)*
*and* Swadhaya *(sacred study of the Divine) be like?*

*What would your practice of* Bhakti Yoga *(devotion) and* Iswara
Pranidhana *(wholehearted dedication to the Divine Light in all)*
*be like?*

*Allow all three to dance together in your life, bringing you to*
*wholeness.*

# THE KLESHAS:
## *Dissolving the Veils*

T HERE ARE FIVE veils that cover the light of the Divine Self, obscuring it from recognition. When we become aware of them, the veils dissolve one by one, and the Divine Light within is seen again.

*Dissolving the five* Kleshas, *or veils, brings forth the radiance of the Divine Self.*

*The five* Kleshas, *or veils, are:*
*Avidya: innocence of our divine nature*
*Asmita: undue trust in the individual self*
*Raga: excessive fondness for fleeting pleasures*
*Dvesa: excessive avoidance of unpleasant experiences*
*Abhinivesah: elusive awareness of immortality*

*Innocence of our divine nature (Avidya) creates a fertile field where the dormant seeds of the other four veils take root.*

*Innocence of our divine nature (Avidya) encourages identification with the ever changing, rather than with the inner stillness of the heart.*

*When undue trust is placed in the individual self (Asmita), it is confused with the Divine Self.*

*Excessive fondness for fleeting pleasures (Raga) causes longing.*

*Excessive avoidance of unpleasant experiences (Dvesa) causes disdain.*

*The elusive awareness of immortality is inherent even for the wise (Abhinivesah).*

*With keen observation and discretion, these Kleshas become translucent.*

*If they have manifested into action, the veils must be dissolved through inward practice.*

II.3 *Dissolving the five* Kleshas, *or veils, brings forth the radiance of the Divine Self.*

> *The five* Kleshas, *or veils, are:*
> Avidya: *innocence of our divine nature*
> Asmita: *undue trust in the individual self*
> Raga: *excessive fondness for fleeting pleasures*
> Dvesa: *excessive avoidance of unpleasant experiences*
> Abhinivesah: *elusive awareness of immortality*

The Divine within is self-effulgent. With the donning of a physical body at birth, certain mental and emotional beliefs materialize as veils. At first these veils are translucent, and the radiant light still shines through. When we look into the eyes of a newborn baby, they reflect the clarity of the resplendent light. As we become increasingly invested in the material world, the seeds of infinite possibilities for wonderful or unkind actions encased in the mind and emotions germinate. The veils thicken and the knowledge that we are Divine Beings fades.

We falsely adopt our fleeting thoughts and emotions as our identity, further occluding the light within. We lose even the memory of its radiance. The belief that we are "merely human" has become our truth.

## KEEP THE LIGHT SHINING BRIGHTLY

Did you ever use a kerosene lamp? At first the light shines bright, illuminating the darkness, enabling us to see clearly. After some time, the glass chimney begins to blacken with soot and the light dims. Turning up the flame only causes the soot to thicken, until the light is totally obscured. Reluctant to clean it earlier, we become obliged to remove the chimney, wash it, and replace it. The yogic practices dissolve the veils in a process similar to cleaning the chimney. With this new clarity, the light shines clear and bright.

*Dissolving the five* Kleshas, *or veils, brings forth the radiance of the Divine Self.*

## II.4 *Innocence of our divine nature* (Avidya) *creates a fertile field where the dormant seeds of the other four veils take root.*

As the veil of innocence envelops our divine nature, the environment becomes conducive to the other four veils deeply rooting. When this essential veil lifts, we behold our divine nature, and the other four veils become powerless.

## II.5 *Innocence of our divine nature* (Avidya) *encourages identification with the ever changing, rather than with the inner stillness of the heart.*

Our lives, hopes, and dreams are built with the conviction that we have some influence over the forces of nature. Often those same hopes and dreams evaporate with the first change in the wind. These changes keep our minds reeling, our hearts in constant hope, and our dreams just out of reach. If we are fortunate enough to realize our dreams, we may after a short time become bored with them as the next castle in the sky forms in our imagination. These dreams are like snowflakes, melting as soon as we take hold of them. Yet day after day we continue to accept triumphs and disappointments as an integral part of the ever-changing nature.

When we turn our view inward, a grand discovery awaits us. Here we find a sacred place where stillness and peace abide, encouraging our hearts to blossom.

This concept is elegantly portrayed in the spiritual practice of turning or whirling practiced by the mystical Middle Eastern order of Sufism. The great Sufi mystic and poet Mevlana Rumi founded the whirling dervishes. Enraptured by the dance of life, the ceremonial turning and whirling inspires even the unbeliever. Arms outstretched in surrender, the left palm pays homage to the earth, the right to heaven. While the left foot is rooted to the world, the right pulses up and down rhythmically to the heart's prayer. The grace and indrawn attention is present in the elegant circular movements. The dance mimics life as the union of constant movement and stillness; all the while the heart stays entwined with the Divine.

Recognizing the Divine within, we dance through the world with joy.

*Innocence of our divine nature* (Avidya) *encourages identification with the ever changing, rather than with the inner stillness of the heart.*

## II.6 *When undue trust is placed in the individual self* (Asmita), *it is confused with the Divine Self.*

Even in the most extraordinary events, the Divine remains anonymous. We accept praise and credit for most of the things we do: "*I* built that"; "*I* healed that person." Do you really believe that you, as an individual self, have the capacity to build something of extraordinary beauty or that you hold the power to heal? This narrow vision of our interaction with the physical world may help to build individual self-esteem, but it fails to capture the ultimate reality.

What happens if your accomplishment is challenged or criticized? Often we become overly upset, terrified to try again.

If, instead, your sense of self-esteem is based on the belief that you are divine, then you will know that all your actions come from that source. Living this way, you will always feel connected to the cosmic dance.

A wise friend reminded me that there were three important words to remember: "no," "yes," and "wow." Try using them in the quantity that the order represents. Use "no" sparingly. It will allow you to have a certain illusory control over your life, but in excess it breeds resistance, fear, and even anger. Overuse of "no" promotes a heaviness and rigidity in your life.

A generous sprinkling of "yes" throughout your life encourages openness and adventure, as it leaves the door open for new possibilities. "Yes" also encourages us to surrender the idea of control and let the heart take over. Life is never dull when you use "yes" frequently.

Saying and thinking "wow" as much as possible will inspire a sense of wonder and gratitude, reminding you of the infinite potential of the Divine Self.

**When undue trust is placed in the individual self (Asmita), *it is confused with the Divine Self*.**

## II.7 *Excessive fondness for fleeting pleasures (Raga) causes longing.*

## II.8  *Excessive avoidance of unpleasant experiences (Dvesa) causes disdain.*

These sutras represent the extremes of the swinging pendulum that tend to overshadow our lives: good and evil, pleasure and pain, love and hate. We tend to think toward the extremes. Actually, there are infinite possibilities between them. Realizing this, we can stop at any one of the midway points and find balance and comfort there. Our hope in practicing Yoga is that our life will stabilize in this way.

Continually striving for the highs, we will probably find that they elude us, and we will feel compelled to climb to steeper and steeper plateaus. We enjoy the thrill of the highest mountain but dislike roaming around in the endless valleys below. Instead, we could be seeking out the endless plain of harmony.

## BUT DID THEY LIVE HAPPILY EVER AFTER?

Having been a monk and a spiritual minister for many years, I find that one of the joys of this vocation is presiding over weddings. On that magical day, each pledges love and dedication to the other. My heart never fails to delight in the splendor of love.

For a growing majority of couples, something changes after the earnestness of the vows. On their wedding day, they've promised to cling to each other for richer or for poorer, in sickness and in health, forsaking all others. Fast-forward several years, and the same two lovebirds have turned into birds of prey. They stand together not at a spiritual altar but at the bar of a court of law. The passion that once fanned the flames of love now swirls the fire of animosity, fueled by wounded feelings and accusations. I often wonder, "What could have caused such a dramatic change?"

If we are used to extremes, we may find ourselves bored when balance and calm come to prevail. When falling in love, at the peak of great passion, it is difficult to remember that there is a valley deep below. Instead of scaling the peaks only to fly off a cliff, ride the peaceful, rolling hills. A balanced relationship promotes growth and liberation for all involved.

*Excessive fondness for fleeting pleasures* (Raga) *causes longing.*

*Excessive avoidance of unpleasant experiences* (Dvesa) *causes disdain.*

The Bhagavad Gita counsels us on the virtues of the middle path: "Peace is granted to those who see the same Self in friend and foe alike, whose mind stays balanced in the midst of honor or dishonor, heat or cold, pleasure or pain, and who maintains equanimity during praise and blame."

The Gita is not advocating avoidance or overindulgence; rather, it points to the mystical path of balance. Often in our zeal for spiritual practices, we feel it is essential to become an ascetic, eliminating the pleasures of the physical world. But in eliminating all the little niceties that make life on the earth fun and enjoyable, we are looking for divinity externally and risk forgetting that what we are seeking is already within us.

## SWEETS MAKE US SWEET

While in India I had the great blessing of being invited to an intimate *satsang* (company of the wise) with Sri Shastraji, a great Yoga master. As he spoke about the Vedas and other such elevated subjects, a plate of tasty treats was placed in front of him. Continuing his discourse, he offered the sweets, encouraging me to take as many as I would like.

He must have noticed my beaming smile as I reached for more than a few. "Ah," he said, "you like sweets?"

"I love sweets!" I said. The great philosopher asked me why.

"Well"—I thought for a moment, reluctantly taking my attention away from the taste sensation in my mouth—"they make me sweet!"

"What a great understanding of the teachings." He chuckled. "The Vedas tell us that when we are able to experience the *sukha* [sweetness or happiness] of life in any form, it serves to remind us of the Divine Self. If we do not experience sweetness, we assume that it is not there. With the absence of *sukha,* our only option is to identify with the opposite, *dukha* [sadness or bitterness]."

Many teachers and translators of the scriptures encourage us to avoid the sweetness in life to better prepare us for the big pay-off, *enlightenment.* It is actually the opposite. When we generously sprinkle our lives with joy and sweetness, their seeds take root within us, reflecting in our every action. This ever-present joy is the greatest enlightenment, and it can be ours right now!

*Excessive fondness for fleeting pleasures* (Raga) *causes longing.*

*Excessive avoidance of unpleasant experiences* (Dvesa) *causes disdain.*

## II.9 *The elusive awareness of immortality is inherent even for the wise* (Abhinivesah).

One of the most vital reasons for spiritual practice is to prepare us for the moment of physical death. Dying can be a time when great apprehension and doubt become our constant companions. Remembering that we are divine and therefore immortal can ease that struggle.

The more we busy ourselves with life's diversions, the less we identify with our bodies' constant wear and tear. Yet our breath betrays us by continuing to count down our allotted time. People diagnosed with life-threatening diseases often have a keener awareness of the "now." They have the grace to know their fate and decide priorities based on a limited engagement on this precious earth. Sometimes it seems their lust for life is stronger than most of ours is, since we delude ourselves into thinking we have an unlimited, noncancelable contract.

The curious way we think of life and death in our society is carved on each gravestone.

NAME

1908–2000

How do you interpret this information? Both dates are very important, the first being when she was born into this world, and the second when she left this world. And the dash? That was the rest of her life! A dash, interesting! It is as if we are born, and we begin to dash to our goal—death. After ninety-two years of running, it seems she finally made it!

We need a reminder *not* to dash. Instead, slow down and appreciate each moment for its beauty and fullness.

*The elusive awareness of immortality is inherent even for the wise* (Abhinivesah).

## A SAINT FOR ALL REASONS

My foremost inspiration from a saintly woman came in the form of Sri Sharada Devi. Most commonly known as the wife of Sri Ramakrishna Paramahansa, she was a luminous teacher in her own right, known to many as the Holy Mother. In her humility the Holy Mother expressed the teachings through her living example.

Often friends or students coming to me during a life crisis did not want to express their emotions, fearing I would find them lacking in "spirituality." In an endeavor to comfort them, I often related one of my favorite teachings from Sri Sharada Devi.

After the death of Sri Ramakrishna, the Holy Mother became the spiritual head (better yet, the spiritual heart!) of the organization. In spite of the fact that the master himself honored her with the position, some of the male monastic disciples doubted that a *woman* could have the spiritual attainment to advise them.

There were, however, a few who recognized her divinity. One young monk who revered her as the Holy Mother personally attended to her needs and served her food with love, devotion, and reverence.

She expected him this particular morning, when another monk appeared with her breakfast. "Where," she asked, "is my *other* dear son?"

"Mother," replied the monk, "I am here to inform you that in the night he left his mortal coil." Immediately on hearing this, tears cascaded down her cheeks. Abandoning herself to grief, she began to sob.

"Mother, how can *you* resort to such emotion? You know that the body is just temporary, that only the soul is immortal. *We are not the body or the mind!*" He had the gall to quote Vedanta (scripture) to her!

With a compassionate smile emanating from her pure heart, she said, "Yes, my son, I know all the sacred teachings. Yet I am still in human form and, therefore, have feelings. Right now my heart is breaking for the physical loss of my beloved son. I honor that pain with my tears."

Within the spiritual traditions, both mind and heart must be honored. Since much emphasis is placed on controlling the mind, it is vital to give the heart its place of honor. It is the guardian to the spark of divinity, the True Self. Be joyful and remember your own immortality.

> I died a mineral and became a plant. I died a plant and rose as an animal.
> I died an animal and I was man [or woman].
> Why should I fear? When was I less by dying?
>
> —*Rumi*

*The elusive awareness of immortality is inherent even for the wise* (Abhinivesah).

## II.10 *With keen observation and discretion, these* Kleshas *become translucent.*

If the veils are present in *feeling and thought,* keen observation is enough to enable us to disperse them.

**With keen observation and discretion, these** Kleshas **become translucent.**

## II.11 *If they have manifested into action, the veils must be dissolved through inward practice.*

When the *Kleshas* manifest in words and actions, their roots are already deep. Mere observation is not enough to displace them. This is the time to call upon the deeper, subtler, and therefore more powerful inner practices. Periods of stillness, introspection, and devotion are summoned to dissolve the veils that hide the inner light.

*If they have manifested into action, the veils must be dissolved through inward practice.*

## EXPERIENCING THE DISSOLVING
## OF THE FIVE *KLESHAS*

*Find a comfortable position, lying down either on the floor or on your bed.*

*Place your right hand on your lower belly and your left hand on your heart.*

*Begin to observe your breath. Is it deep and regular? Shallow and irregular?*

*Shift your attention to the idea that breath propels life.*

*Each time you inhale, there is an inflow of life's energy entering your body.*

*With the exhalation observe the energy leaving your body.*

*This is followed by a moment's hesitation, a space between the two breaths and between the two worlds.*

*Notice any discomfort in your body, emotions, or mind.*

*Continue for a few minutes. Invoke the attitude of gratitude for this life-giving breath.*

*Now, gradually, shift your attention to the center of your heart and the light that dwells within, the Divine Self.*

*Can you begin to experience the light of the Divine Self?*

*Be still and patient until you feel the veils thinning.*

*Can you identify any aspect of your belief system that keeps the veil of innocence (Avidya) in place?*

*Once you have identified it, can you envision a symbol, a feeling, or a word that can return you to the light of the Divine?*

*Breathe deeply, enhancing the energy and spreading the light through the body, mind, and emotions, coming back to full consciousness.*

*Tuck the memory of this experience deep into the recesses of your heart and sprinkle it liberally throughout your day.*

*After some time, and with continual practice, you will find the veils become more and more transparent.*

*As the Divine Light radiates through us, it illuminates who we are, shedding light on all we do.*

# KARMA AND *KARMA YOGA:*
## *As You Sow, So You Shall Reap*

THESE SUTRAS ATTEMPT to explain the intricate aspects of karma, the cycle of actions seeding other actions. Its concept is widely known, and often quite misunderstood. Hopefully, this commentary will alleviate some of the confusion and allow you to understand the basic principles and intent of karma.

*The womb of karma (Karmasala), sheathed by the* Kleshas *(veils), gives birth to experiences now and in the future.*

*As long as the veils encase the womb of karma (Karmasala), all actions will be affected.*

*Karma bears fruits according to the type and quality of the seed planted and the care given to its growth.*

II.12 *The womb of karma (Karmasala), sheathed by the Kleshas (veils), gives birth to experiences now and in the future.*

II.13 *As long as the veils encase the womb of karma (Karmasala), all actions will be affected.*

II.14 *Karma bears fruits according to the type and quality of the seed planted and the care given to its growth.*

Karma is popularly understood as a kind of universal punishment for our sins and a reward for our good deeds. This simplistic definition is reinforced by the notion of someone or something far above us passing judgment and sentencing us. So when bad things happen to good people, we are outraged at the unfairness of life and question the sanity of this higher judge.

The concept of karma depicted in the Yoga Sutras and the Bhagavad Gita is in fact a neutral energy that, when activated by the mind and emotions, manifests into action. This action leads to a reaction that in turn spawns new action and continues the cycle. It is our choice, though not always a conscious one, whether to move karma into fruition or let it remain dormant. While most of us choose to believe that the actions of others have the greatest effect on us, it is actually our own deeds that have the most profound influence.

The idea of blame or judgment is removed if we understand that our karma is directly affected by the density of the veils (*Kleshas*) that cloak our divine nature. When filtered through opaque layers, the inner light appears dim and distorted. This significantly alters our motives and our actions. Unable to easily identify with our true nature, we think and act for material gain. This is what turns the constantly spinning wheel of action and reaction that drives us day after day, month after month, life after life.

Looking at the world from a dualistic view, we eagerly polarize karma into good or bad, white or black. Instead, when we view it as a rainbow of colors, each karma brings us a message to shape our lives.

Karma is similar to the energy of an electrical current. The outlet in your house supplies needed electricity. Is that good or bad? If you plug in a lamp and receive light, you might say, "Ah! Electricity is good. I have good karma; there is light to read at night." However, if you stick your finger into that same outlet and get a shock, you might think, "Ah! Electricity is bad! What bad karma I must have to get shocked in my own home." Electricity, like karma, is neither good nor bad; its effect is determined by how we treat it.

Individual karmas become our teachers, encouraging us to remember the True Self. When a few join together for a larger lesson, the consequences often seem disproportionate to the minor event that gave birth to them. It is those times that reinforce our belief that karma is either bad or good. In fact, it is just a bigger lesson for us to learn.

## THE FRUITS RIPEN IN THREE WAYS

Managing our karma is like planting and tending a garden. Before planting any garden, we first must realistically consider what plants grow well in the particular soil and climate. Each plant or tree, depending on the conditions, has the potential to produce delicious fruits or inedible ones. We must use our best judgment as to which seeds to plant and which plants to nourish.

Three types of karma emerge from the womb of karma (*Karma-sala*) into our garden: *Parabda, Agami,* and *Sangita.*

*Parabda* is the karma generated from past actions that affect the present. It governs those actions that are already determined and cannot be changed, such as where and when you were born, who your birth parents are, and so on. You may wish you could change these events, but it is not possible. The trees planted long before are now bearing fruit. It is too late to change the type of fruit *or* the taste.

*Agami* karma is generated as the fruits of present actions take hold in future actions. This gives us time to make changes, but only if we act promptly. Careful consideration must be taken before planting. Having prepared the soil and gathered seedlings from a sweet apple, we lovingly place them in the earth. We know that we will be rewarded with a great harvest if each plant receives the optimal amount of water, sun, and room to grow. We carefully eliminate those plants that spring up to threaten the delicate seedlings. When we plant and weed with discrimination and compassion, the plants we are caring for will thrive. Likewise, the karmas we are planting now bear fruit in the future.

If we plant a peach seed, it would be unrealistic to expect to come back after a few years and pick apples. If at the time of planting, the seeds were inferior, or the tree was not well tended, the fruit will reflect those conditions. We may not be able to change the quality of the fruits; we can, however, change our attitude toward them. Instead of chiding a tree for producing sour apples, the creative solution would be to add a little sweetener and make an apple pie!

You might have heard a friend say something to this effect: "My fiancé is not very kind to me. Maybe *after* we get married, his attitude will change." Expecting someone to change is a dangerous notion. This is the time to nip *Agami* karma in the bud. A well-considered decision not to marry this person can eliminate heartache in the future.

*Sangita* karma keeps the seeds safe within the *Karmasala*. They are yet unsprouted. Assessing whether to plant the seeds of karma, we recall certain life experiences and plant with caution, knowing that once the seeds germinate, we reap the harvest. Even if we try to pull them up, the roots have grown deep, and the underground growth may continue. It is best to honor our intuition regarding which of the incubating seeds we plant.

Your choices may sound something like this. "This situation reminds me of the time I stayed in that job because it paid well, even though it made me miserable. Now that a similar situation has come up, I was almost fooled into doing the same thing again. But I caught myself in time."

We are not alone in our karma. Each person we meet has some influence on how our karma plays out. When you are single, your karma is entwined with that of your friends and family. If you marry, you now have your karma, your spouse's karma, and your combined karma, not to mention children, in-laws, grandchildren, and so many others. The winds of change scatter our karmic seeds far and wide.

Innumerable seeds from this life and previous ones are housed in the *Karmasala,* and it may seem that many of them come to fruition at once. We have accumulated needs for action or reaction—karmas— from all our choices in this life. If this seems overwhelming, it may be helpful to stretch our concept of mortality to understand that we, as souls, will incarnate many times to fulfill the many karmas.

*The womb of karma* (Karmasala), *sheathed by the* Kleshas (veils), *gives birth to experiences now and in the future.*

*As long as the veils encase the womb of karma* (Karmasala), *all actions will be affected.*

*Karma bears fruits according to the type and quality of the seed planted and the care given to its growth.*

## HOW THE *GUNAS* (ATTRIBUTES OF NATURE) INTERPLAY WITH KARMA

No one is free of action (karma) even for a moment,
because each is helplessly moved by the *gunas.*
—Bhagavad Gita

The ever-present *gunas* (attributes of nature) are forces that influence not only our karma but also our attitude toward it. If we are able to recognize and transcend the *gunas,* karma will be affected less.

Enmeshed in the *Tamasic,* or static, *guna,* we may be blind to the cause of our circumstances. We hold the attitude then that we can do anything we want without suffering the consequences. This blindness can inadvertently create more karma.

A teenager's wild driving is spurred on by her inability to imagine losing control of the tremendous machine she is manipulating. A benign near miss might cause her arrogance to retreat, but a boomerang effect can cause the *Tamas* to deepen, presenting fear and immobility. The balance point of *Sattwa* is not even in view.

If we are steeped in the *Rajasic guna,* we are constantly irritated by how unfair life is, believing we deserve better. Sometimes, gloating when good things happen to us, we ignore the circumstances or feelings of others. When we are immersed in *Rajas,* we tend to not share our good fortune, and this brings more karma upon us.

When overly *Rajasic* people are diagnosed with a disease, they may become upset and feel victimized. This anger, diverted into righteous indignation, can prompt them to speak out against the unfair healthcare system, or they may start a class-action suit against a company for misleading the public. These actions may not eradicate their karma on the disease level but certainly can help them and others not to create any more karma in this arena.

A moment's hesitation in anger will save a hundred days of sorrow.

—*Chinese proverb*

When we abide predominately with the *Sattwic guna*, we accept with equanimity any and all karmas that come, realizing they are blessings in disguise. If, unexpectedly, we were to receive a large amount of money, our immediate response would be to share it with those in need. When negative circumstances befall us, we understand they come from seeds planted long before. Acceptance allows us to soothe the reaction to this karma, thwarting any need to make others suffer. We can feel that, by contributing to another's pain, we are not relieved; instead, our own suffering intensifies. With the grace of compassion, we understand the suffering of others. If we are able to metaphorically "walk a mile in another's moccasins," we may actually feel blessed by our karma.

Whenever someone complained about life's woes, my mother would say, "Take your troubles and put them in the center of a circle with all the other troubles in the world. Examine them all. I bet you will be grateful to choose yours once again."

*The womb of karma* (Karmasala), *sheathed by the* Kleshas *(veils), gives birth to experiences now and in the future.*

*As long as the veils encase the womb of karma* (Karmasala), *all actions will be affected.*

*Karma bears fruits according to the type and quality of the seed planted and the care given to its growth.*

## TRANSFORMING KARMA

Looking through the teachings of the Old and New Testaments, we find karma apparent in many sections. One of the most notable is "an eye for an eye and a tooth for a tooth." It seems that thousands of years later we are still battling, plotting our revenge, or trying to get even with something or someone, making it our duty not to let anyone get away with anything.

Asked about the adage, the Reverend Martin Luther King Jr. mused, that if we follow the words of the Old Testament *exactly,* and take an eye for an eye and a tooth for a tooth, we will all become *blind and toothless.*

Constantly plagued by the mounting annoyances of everyday life, we are able to use the myriad Yoga practices to connect with the *Sattwic* aspect of our nature. Challenging as it might be, after some time the mind and emotions will acquiesce to calmness rather than aggravation.

> Whatever greatness a person does is followed by others who set their values by her/his example. They will not disturb others who may be still attached to the fruits of their actions. By continually performing selfless actions, the wise person influences others in all they do.
>
> —Bhagavad Gita

*The womb of karma* (Karmasala), *sheathed by the* Kleshas *(veils), gives birth to experiences now and in the future.*

*As long as the veils encase the womb of karma* (Karmasala), *all actions will be affected.*

*Karma bears fruits according to the type and quality of the seed planted and the care given to its growth.*

## TRANSFORMING KARMA THROUGH *KARMA YOGA*

If action is inevitable, how can we circumvent the need for reaction and prevent more karma from accruing? Can we slow down the ever-spinning wheel? The secret is *Karma Yoga* or *Seva* (selfless service).

*Karma Yoga* tempers the law of karma (action and its subsequent reaction) by redirecting the effects of our actions through selfless service. If we must reap what we sow, let us sow seeds of a sweet and tasty fruit.

There are as many ways to serve as people to be served. *Karma Yoga* is about doing our best, not expecting praise or blame. To do the deed for the sake of doing, not looking for the reward, is at the heart of *Karma Yoga*. We may feel gratified in seeing others happy, but let this be a side effect, not the main goal.

One thing I know: The only ones among you who will be really happy are those who will have sought and found how to serve.

—*Albert Schweitzer*

Before we can begin to give selflessly, our hearts must open to be able to recognize other people's needs. We then honor them by listening to what they need, and by providing what they ask rather than our opinion of it. As our hearts open further, we serve them without judgment, bathing them in compassion, allowing their dignity to be preserved. This kind of giving benefits both giver and receiver. In *Karma Yoga* we may perform the same duties and actions as before, but now our zeal is increased, just by letting go of expectations and results. For a little extra power, bring in the *Bhakti* (devotional) aspect and envision you are dedicating your actions to the Divine.

Every spiritual tradition encourages service as a way to purify the heart. To embark on your path of service, there are many repu-

table organizations you can participate in and support. In the beginning you may feel the desire to be recognized for your service:
a thank-you letter, your name on a plaque, something of the sort.
Giving anonymously can help limit this attachment. Also, at first
you may feel more comfortable giving money than hands-on service. Slowly begin to give more of yourself and notice how it affects
the rest of your life.

> Letting go of attachment to the fruits of one's actions, one is ever
> content and does not have needs. Though one appears to be doing
> things (karma), actually the higher Self is the doer.
>
> —Bhagavad Gita

We all carry impressions (*Samskaras*) from birth, early childhood, and even other lifetimes. The type of *Karma Yoga* you choose
can help you to reduce the effects of any traumas and encourage
healing. If you came from a poor family and are now financially
comfortable, feeding people or donating clothing can make your
heart sing. If you lost a parent at a young age, becoming part of a
Big Sister program mentoring a young girl will be your joy. Customize *Karma Yoga* to your particular passion.

The Serenity Prayer seems to beautifully explain karma: "May I
find the serenity to accept the things that cannot be changed, the
courage to change the things that I can, and the wisdom to know
the difference."

> Never doubt that a small group of thoughtful, committed citizens can
> change the world. Indeed, it is the only thing that ever has.
>
> —Margaret Mead

*The womb of karma* (Karmasala), *sheathed by the* Kleshas
*(veils), gives birth to experiences now and in the future.*

*As long as the veils encase the womb of karma (Karmasala), all actions will be affected.*

*Karma bears fruits according to the type and quality of the seed planted and the care given to its growth.*

## THE RIGHT LIVELIHOOD—DOES MONEY MOO?

"What about my work?" you may be thinking. "I need to earn a livelihood. I have a family to support! I cannot afford to donate *all my time!*"

Choose a job you love and you will never have to work a day in your life.
—*Unknown*

Whatever service you perform in the world, let it be compatible with your spiritual path. If you sacrifice your inner convictions for the sake of money, you will always feel in debt, no matter what your bank balance may be. Even if your service in the world is not directly connected to your practice, unite it by serving all with a full heart.

The monetary compensation you receive carries the vibration of the work you do. For example, if you are a vegetarian for reasons of *Ahimsa* (reverence for all life) and take a job selling meat in some way, you may find the lack of alignment unsettling. If out of necessity you *must* do that type of work, with each portion served, send a blessing to the animal's spirit. This will infuse the action with awareness and gratitude, allowing you to feel more at peace in your heart. If the contradiction continues to gnaw at you despite your best efforts, a change of profession may be necessary.

A poignant lesson was given to me during the time our ashram was building LOTUS (Light of Truth Universal Shrine), an ecumenical shrine. As people would hear of the great endeavor to unite all religions under one holy roof, they would become inspired and want to donate. Some would come to give of their time; others would leave a monetary donation. After visiting for a few days, one very wealthy man resonated with what was taking place and handed Sri Swamiji a check for a sizable donation. With a look of pleasant surprise, Sri Swamiji asked what the man did to earn such money. A bit shyly the man said, "Well, Swamiji, actually I am a cattle rancher."

"So" said Swamiji, "you make your money raising cows and then sending them to the slaughterhouse?" The man replied that he did.

Handing the man back his check, Swamiji told him, "You are always welcome to come and stay with us. But we cannot accept your money. It cries MOOO!"

Even something as subtle as what type of stock or bond you invest in affects you. If you keep your money in a bank and it earns interest, how is the bank investing that money? There are now socially responsible mutual funds that do not invest in weapons, alcohol, cigarettes, and so on. How you earn and invest your livelihood reverberates in everything it buys. Take time to know the company (*satsang*) your money is keeping. Earn it wisely.

When you perform an action, any action, offer *all result*s to the highest good, and know that the deed will reverberate throughout your life. When you keep your heart in service, you can trust that all your needs will be cared for.

## *KARMA YOGA* AND YOU

During these busy times, most of us consider it a luxury to take time to retreat from the world to the spirit, and it is touted as a blessing for the few. This is great *Karma Yoga* for us. When we feel nurtured, it is easy to nurture others. When we do not nurture ourselves, we are unable to draw upon qualities of love, faith, and other spiritual virtues. Not paying attention to our own needs causes them to burrow and hide deep within our hearts.

*Karma Yoga* for yourself can be even fifteen minutes to one hour a day. If you do it regularly, that short period of time is enough to revitalize body, mind, and emotions and lead you home to the spirit.

Always give from the overflow of your well, not from its depth.

—*Sufi saying*

The good news is that Golden Age consciousness is ripening right now. Many are acknowledging their spirituality and allowing it to blossom. With this rising group consciousness, the wheel of karma becomes a spiral that elevates us upward from the Iron Age to the Golden Age.

When the heart and spirit are held supreme, the Golden Age is now!

*The womb of karma* (Karmasala), *sheathed by the* Kleshas *(veils), gives birth to experiences now and in the future.*

*As long as the veils encase the womb of karma (Karmasala), all actions will be affected.*

*Karma bears fruits according to the type and quality of the seed planted and the care given to its growth.*

## EXPERIENCING A PAST KARMA THAT HAS A DIRECT EFFECT ON THE PRESENT

*Remember a significant event in your life. You or someone else could have initiated it. Can you trace the experience of that occurrence and how it affected the next related incident? Do either of the original actions have reverberations even to the present?*

*It could be a teacher encouraging you to go on to college. Had she not handed you the college application along with papers for a scholarship, you might not have thought to apply for the monetary allotment. Because of her kindness, you were able to go to college and then law school, which allowed you years later to become a senator.*

*Go now the other way. Take an event in your life now and trace it back to when it was seeded. If the seed could be exchanged or replanted, how would it look different?*

*Next time you begin to do a significant action, think how the chain of events evolving from it will influence your life. You still have time to change it!*

## EXPERIENCING THE BLESSINGS OF *KARMA YOGA* (SELFLESS SERVICE) FOR OTHERS

*Choose an aspect of service that you would like to offer. It could be for an individual or through an organization.*

*If at first you would like to donate money, that is a great start toward opening the heart. As time goes on, involve yourself more and more, finding a place to offer your goodwill that fits with your particular temperament.*

*Start to block off time regularly, on a weekly or monthly basis, for the service. Notice the excuses that come to keep you from doing it.*

*Convincing yourself to do the Seva (service), your heart begins to open. After a while you may find yourself canceling other events to enable you to do Karma Yoga! You soon begin to experience that the small amount you give is paled by the great joy you receive. Notice if the hurdles in your life become more relaxed.*

## EXPERIENCING THE BLESSINGS OF *KARMA YOGA* (SELFLESS SERVICE) FOR YOURSELF

*In the midst of the busyness of life, find what feeds and nurtures you. In order for us to give lovingly to others, we need to feel the Divine within.*

*If your body is sore or aching, a luxurious bubble bath or a relaxing massage, even an extra couple of minutes in deep relaxation, can be profoundly healing. A sweet lie-down in the middle of the afternoon can feel like a week at the spa.*

*If it is the mind and emotions that pain you, remember to give them something fun to do, not always serious thoughts and feelings. Read a light and inspiring book, see a romantic comedy (that has nothing to do with your own relationship), do that art project you have been putting off, or just watch the simplicity of rain.*

*When you remember to serve yourself first, the service to others flows forth.*

*Make* Karma Yoga *a steady habit. It encourages the wheel of karma, instead of spinning in a continuous circle, to spiral upward, taking you to the joy of your true nature.*

# JNANA YOGA:
## The Yoga of Intuitive Wisdom

HERE WE ARE introduced to the subtle power of Intuitive Wisdom, the grand wisdom of *Jnana Yoga*.

These sutras are positioned at the seam of the physical and spiritual worlds. They perch us on the threshold of *Asthaanga Yoga* (the Eight-Faceted Path), where prudent insights are offered to sustain this pristine wisdom.

*Intuitive Wisdom empowers us to expand beyond the constantly changing natural world (seen) to the abode of the Divine Spirit (seer).*

*With this understanding, once-vital difficulties become impotent.*

*The source of these difficulties is the inability to recognize the Divine Spirit (seer) as omniscient and therefore separate from the constantly changing natural world (seen).*

*When understood as illusory (Maya), nature (seen) and her attributes the* gunas *exist to serve the Divine Self (seer) with both enjoyment and liberation.*

*These attributes of nature (gunas) are both tangible and intangible.*

*The Divine Self (seer) observes the world without being affected by it.*

*The natural world (seen) exists for the benefit of the Divine Self (seer).*

*With realization of the Divine Self (seer), the illusory natural world (seen) becomes transparent, though still seemingly very real to those enmeshed in it.*

*When the Divine Self (seer) and nature (seen) unite, this dynamic and powerful synergy creates the illusory world, obscuring the vision of spirit.*

*This union is consummated when we forget the Divine Self (seer).*

*With constant remembrance of the Divine Self, no such union is possible.*

*Established in the grace of Intuitive Wisdom, we experience liberation.*

*Liberation is recognized in seven ways: we no longer feel the need for knowledge, to stay away from anything or anyone, to gather material things, or to act, and our constant companions are joy, faith, and clarity.*

II.15 *Intuitive Wisdom empowers us to expand beyond the constantly changing natural world (seen) to the abode of the Divine Spirit (seer).*

As our consciousness expands, we realize that there is an essential difference between the inner world of the spirit and the outer world of nature. An Intuitive Wisdom emerges, strengthened by constant acknowledgment. Our intuition whispers to us in a voice that is often overshadowed by the louder, more prominent voice of our thoughts. It is the quiet voice of our spirit guiding us toward the light. That Intuitive Wisdom is always to be trusted, as it springs from the gratitude of knowing. It cannot be influenced by messages of this changing world; rather, it is rooted in unchanging reality.

Elisabeth Kübler-Ross, a noble pioneer in the field of end-of-life care, was often asked if she believed in reincarnation. Her quick-witted reply was "I do not believe in reincarnation—I know it to be true!"

As our intuition develops, the perception that our life is formed from outside influences is welcomingly transformed, and we gain the knowledge that the True Self is the primary influence. All tangible world experiences are delivered by our senses and interpreted by our thoughts and emotions. That which is material is temporary and causes us to regret its passing. We understand that the world does not have the capacity to secure our everlasting happiness. The more we understand the complexity of nature's effect on us, the more effortlessly we are able to expand beyond her grasp and align with our true knowledge.

When we are able to know the Self, all else is known.
—Bhagavad Gita

## WISDOM FROM THE HEART

Most often *Jnana Yoga* is described from a purely mental perspective using terms like "reason," "discernment," and "discrimination." These words are fitting if we are addressing wisdom only from the mental perspective. Wisdom also comes from the heart, as intuition.

Directing our lives from our Intuitive Wisdom, nothing is deemed good or bad. We are simply able to observe where the tossing *gunas* have temporarily lit. We may find we are happy to see a friend one minute, unhappy to see her the next. All this has to do with the way the mind and emotions are playing out at that very moment. The effects of past conditions can cause strong reactions if we are not vigilant. *Patterns are difficult to change.* As we recognize the True Self, everything else in the world becomes secondary. Any desire to possess or run from the world is dissipated. Instead in our stillness it comes to us.

When you understand the physical world, there is nothing to hinder you from playing and having fun with everything. At first it may seem overwhelming to experience the world in this unusual way, but like any other skill you learn, the ease and joy come as you become more proficient.

When you were young, were you afraid to ride a bike? "How could I possibly balance on those thin tires? How do I steer, and more importantly, how do I stop?" In the beginning you had to use training wheels while someone vigilantly held on to your bicycle's seat. After a while the training wheels were removed, but that attentive protector still held firmly on to your seat, until finally one day, although you were shaky, you rode alone. That was many years ago and not even a whisper of doubt joins you as you now mount your bike. Only the freedom and joy remain, making the whole world your playground.

The real power comes when we can expand beyond the constant changes in nature and be firmly grounded in our Intuitive Wisdom.

*Intuitive Wisdom empowers us to expand beyond the constantly changing natural world (seen) to the abode of the Divine Spirit (seer).*

II.16 *With this understanding, once-vital difficulties become impotent.*

II.17 *The source of these difficulties is the inability to recognize the Divine Spirit (seer) as omniscient and therefore separate from the constantly changing natural world (seen).*

II.18 *When understood as illusory (Maya), nature (seen) and her attributes the gunas exist to serve the Divine Self (seer) with both enjoyment and liberation.*

Here Yoga wisdom introduces us to two distinct aspects: the one who *sees* (the True Self) and that which is *seen* (everything else). Most of the time we identify with what is *seen* rather than with the one who sees. Difficulties manifest because we do not understand that everything in this natural world changes and cannot be slowed, halted, or possessed. The *only thing we can hold on to* is the knowledge of the True Self.

Once upon a time there was a great queen. Graced by realizing the eternal truth that ultimately she could not possess anything, she decided to free all her possessions. She issued a proclamation to the entire principality, offering her worldly goods to anyone who wanted them. The only restriction was that the treasures could not leave the palace until after the stroke of five o'clock on the appointed day.

It was 4:55 on the day of this great giveaway, and all were eagerly standing by their selected prizes. A strange and imposing woman entered the palace. The queen greeted her and immediately apologized because everything of value had already been claimed. This did not faze the woman in the least; just before the stroke of five, she took her place next to the queen and inquired calmly, "Your Majesty, when you said *everything* in the palace was to be given away, did that also include *you*?"

Surprised and bewildered, the queen stammered, "I did say *everything*; I guess that means me too." Then the woman said boldly, "I choose *you*!" "But why," stammered the queen, "would you want *me*? I am now penniless." Embracing the queen at the exact stroke of five, the woman proclaimed, "Everyone *stop* where you are! No one is to leave the palace until all the treasures are returned to their rightful places." Laughing, she continued to enlighten the people, "You went for the small trinkets, but *I* have chosen the greatest treasure of all, the queen. Because when I possess *her*, I possess *everything*!"

It is not only the material possessions that we want to hold on to but also the desire for our bodies and minds to either stay the same or be different from what they are. When we are young, we want to look and act grown up. When we are graying, we add color so we can look younger. Once we realize that everything in nature changes, we liberate ourselves from wanting things to be different than they actually are. We enjoy every moment.

An interesting way to observe this phenomenon is to browse through a photo album that captures you from childhood up to the present day. Start at the beginning and try to remember how you felt and thought at that moment in time. You may not remember as far back as infancy, but notice at what age the memories start. Then progressively go through the photos, noting how you felt at those frozen moments in your story. Observe the snapshots of yourself on your first day at school or at a ballet lesson. Even though your body size was smaller and your wants and needs may have differed, isn't there something deep inside you that feels the same? Can you detect a similar awareness weaving through your entire life? There is an interior sameness that never changes, a presence watching, guiding us; it is our *Intuitive Wisdom*.

I remember my mother at age ninety-one emphatically calling me to her room. "Look," she said, gesturing to the mirror. I looked but was unable to discern what the surprising discovery was. "There." She pointed. "Who is that old woman looking back at me? It can't be me. I'm not that old, am I?"

It does seem to happen so fast. One day we are playing grown-up wearing our mother's high heels, then at what seems like the next moment, *our children* are playing grown-up with *our* things. That is the temperament of the changing world: The only constancy is within.

If we trust our Intuitive Wisdom, everything can be enjoyable because we have found the magic wand to convert everything that life brings into joy.

*With this understanding, once-vital difficulties become impotent.*

*The source of these difficulties is the inability to recognize the Divine Spirit (seer) as omniscient and therefore separate from the constantly changing natural world (seen).*

*When understood as illusory (Maya), nature (seen) and her attributes the* gunas *exist to serve the Divine Self (seer) with both enjoyment and liberation.*

II.19 *These attributes of nature* (gunas) *are both tangible and intangible.*

There are various stages to the manifestation of the *gunas*. Some are apparent as our senses inform us how things are now and how they then change. We are less aware of the intangible changes. Most of us have not developed the resources to grasp that which we are unable to know with the senses. As we develop our inner perception, we are able to know that we know what there is to know.

When nature began, it was indefinite and without expression. From this stage the *gunas* (attributes of nature) formed and were in balance. As the universe evolved, the *gunas* began to shift dominance, and the world as we know it came into being. The *buddhi* (intellect), *ahamkara* (thoughts and emotions), and *manas* (senses) that we spoke about earlier manifested from the disproportionate interplay of the *gunas*.

In a way it is like baking bread. First we have the idea of bread and how it will taste and how to make it. Next is actually gathering the ingredients, which vary in quantity according to the type of bread we are baking. Then we mix the individual measured ingredients together until they form dough ready to be kneaded. Sometimes we must add more flour or water to make the consistency just right. It then is allowed to rise, before being baked in the oven. Only when the bread is in its totally manifested state (baked and cooled) do we employ our senses to eat and enjoy it.

**These attributes of nature (gunas) *are both tangible and intangible*.**


**II.20** *The Divine Self (seer) observes the world without being affected by it.*

**II.21** *The natural world (seen) exists for the benefit of the Divine Self (seer).*

II.22 *With realization of the Divine Self (seer), the illusory natural world (seen) becomes transparent, though still seemingly very real to those enmeshed in it.*

II.23 *When the Divine Self (seer) and nature (seen) unite, this dynamic and powerful synergy creates the illusory world, obscuring the vision of spirit.*

II.24 *This union is consummated when we forget the Divine Self (seer).*

II.25 *With constant remembrance of the Divine Self, no such union is possible.*

At this point you may be wondering, "If life could be simpler if we kept our awareness on the Divine Self, why are we not designed to do that?" We *are designed* to make the decision where to direct our awareness. But most of us choose to keep it focused on the material world, perpetuating the *grand illusion (Maha Maya)* of life. However, it is only an illusion to those who understand that it is an illusion. To the rest, it seems *very real.*

## AWAKING FROM THE DREAM

Illusion (*Maya*) in this sense is like a waking dream. While we are dreaming (either during the day or night), it *appears* to be very real. Measuring a person's physiological responses during an active dream state reveals that the blood pressure rises along with the heart rate. The eyes dart back and forth; sometimes the legs and

arms move as if running. If you sleep with another person, you may
have even gotten kicked or poked during one of their very active
dreams.

Most of the time when we awaken, we quickly become aware
that we had been dreaming. Other times, though, we are *unable*
to differentiate the dream state from the waking state. If it is a
wonderful dream, we do not want to let go of it; in other cases,
as much as we want to awaken from it, an unhappy dream creeps
into our waking state. This is the way of *Maya*. Unless we are able
to completely wake up our consciousness, we constantly dwell in
a waking dream. When we do experience enlightenment, we wake
up and realize it was all an illusion, unreal.

This morning you may have looked outside and said, "I do not
want to go for a walk today; the sun is not shining." At midnight
you might doubt the existence of the sun, since it is nowhere to be
seen. In our minds we all know that the sun is always there, even
though sometimes it is engulfed by clouds or on the other side of
the earth from us. Even when the sun is hidden, it remains the
life-giving force that sustains our physical existence. In the same
way, our True Self transmits life force to the body, mind, and emotions, but because we cannot *see* the True Self or *experience* it as
real, we doubt its existence.

## PLAYING THE FOOL

Mullah Nasrudin was a great Sufi mystic whose method of teaching was to play the part of the fool. (He *purposely* played that part!)
One fine day one of his disciples questioned him, "Oh, great mullah, which is more important: the sun or the moon?"

He answered without hesitation, "The moon, of course. During
the day the sun is not so important because there is already light.

But at night the moon is vital because it is our only source of light."
He tried to trick them into thinking that the moon is self-effulgent
like the sun, not merely the reflection of the sun's rays. Can we
trick ourselves into remembering that our thoughts, emotions, and
intellect are not self-effulgent but merely a reflection? They are
reflections that come from either the external material world or the
light within. Often it is difficult to discern their origin.

Much of the time our identity is molded by who *we think we
are* and by the feedback we receive from others, rather than by the
eternal light. As we cultivate our Intuitive Wisdom, the light of the
Self clearly and brightly influences all dimensions of us. In this
elevated consciousness, when you are unhappy, *you know* you are
unhappy; when you are happy, *you know* you are happy. You then
become the knower in all conditions. And nature is here to help us
become liberated.

*The Divine Self (seer) observes the world without being affected
by it.*

*The natural world (seen) exists for the benefit of the Divine Self
(seer).*

*With realization of the Divine Self (seer), the illusory natural
world (seen) becomes transparent, though still seemingly very
real to those enmeshed in it.*

*When the Divine Self (seer) and nature (seen) unite, this
dynamic and powerful synergy creates the illusory world,
obscuring the vision of spirit.*

*This union is consummated when we forget the Divine Self
(seer).*

*With constant remembrance of the Divine Self, no such union is possible.*

## II.26 *Established in the grace of Intuitive Wisdom, we experience liberation.*

This is the key to freedom. By constant observation through Intuitive Wisdom, we know that we are the eternal unchanging Self. If spirit (seer) and nature (seen) give us opposite experiences, we are able to recognize the Self (seer) only through the depth of our Intuitive Wisdom and knowledge. When they unite for the purpose of freedom, nature (seen) helps us to find and reflect the eternal Self (seer).

Whatever you think, so you become. If you believe you are limited, you will be limited; if you believe you are free, you are free.

There is a wonderful strategy that is used to train an elephant to stay in one place. At an early age, the elephant has a large, thick chain attached to her foot. If she tries to stray, the strong chain gives the signal to go no farther. As the baby elephant grows in strength, a large rope replaces the heavy chain. The tether continues to *decrease* in size and strength until the elephant is fully grown.

This may seem counterintuitive, but it is not possible to find a chain or rope strong enough to restrain the huge adult animal. With this training, though, a small cord does the job. Because her memory holds the experience of being restricted by a chain stronger than her baby muscles could resist, the grown elephant assumes that the small cord continues to bind her.

How many tethers are still holding us attached to our minds and emotions?

Through constant observation, the distinction between the changing qualities of what is perceived and the unchanging quality of what perceives becomes evident.

The man [or woman] who has no inner life is the slave of his [or her] surroundings.

—Henri Frédéric Amiel

*Established in the grace of Intuitive Wisdom, we experience liberation.*

II.27 *Liberation is recognized in seven ways: we no longer feel the need for knowledge, to stay away from anything or anyone, to gather material things, or to act, and our constant companions are joy, faith, and clarity.*

There are different ways to interpret the various wisdom paths to freedom. Some view it as gradual, as if experiencing the dawn, where each moment the magnitude of the light becomes greater and greater, until it is seen in its totality. With this view our longing for material things and even our thirst for knowledge dwindle in the promising presence of the eternal. Along with the light there is an ever-quickening dawning of joy, faith, and clarity. (This is considered the *Bhakti* [devotional] way to enlightenment.)

The other way is not gradual; rather, it suggests that after all the practices have aligned, consciousness spontaneously illuminates. This view is more reminiscent of turning on a light switch than of a gradual dawning. It holds the same yearnings, and through willpower it encourages the casting away of material effects that impede the way. (This is considered the *Jnani* way to enlightenment.)

While there are many who tout *Jnana Yoga* as a direct and expedient way to merge with eternal light, it seems to be a matter of temperament. Both are tried-and-true paths to the Divine. Embrace whatever avenue you feel most in tune with; there are always benefits to balance in both.

## A *JNANI,* A *BHAKTI,* AND A PILE OF PEANUTS

Observe two people eating peanuts. Can you distinguish the *Jnani* (student of Intuitive Wisdom) from the *Bhakti* (devotee)? The first one cracks the shell and immediately pops the sweet kernel into her mouth, delighting in the taste before going on to the next nut. The other person unshells the nut and carefully places it in a pile, saving the delicacy for the time when all the nuts are ready.

The first person has the personality more fitting a *Bhakti* because she wants to taste the sweetness all the way through the process. The second person, not wanting to be distracted from her mission, looks forward to eating the whole pile after accomplishing the unsheathing and sorting. The *Bhakti* is similar to the dawning light and the *Jnani* is more like the light switch. The result is the same: They remember they are one with the Divine Self.

> Beholding the Self by the Self, one is satisfied in the Self.
>
> —Bhagavad Gita

Having written all this about *Jnana Yoga,* I urge you to resist the temptation to get *too* caught up in esoteric philosophy. While it is important to know why we are doing the practices, it can also be a way of corralling us toward intellectual gymnastics, leaving the True Self still occluded. *Philosophy without practice is ineffective; practice without philosophy is precarious.* Asthaanga Yoga, the eight-faceted path that follows, offers practices that bring the *Jnana Yoga* sutras into our daily life.

*Liberation is recognized in seven ways: we no longer feel the need for knowledge, to stay away from anything or anyone, to gather material things, or to act, and our constant companions are joy, faith, and clarity.*

## EXPERIENCING WHO YOU ARE BY KNOWING WHAT YOU ARE NOT

*Have the body in a comfortable position, spine erect, shoulders relaxed. Begin to observe the body. Check to see if everything is relaxed—your toes, feet, ankles, shins, calves, knees, thighs, hips, hands, wrists, forearms, etc.*

*Inhale through the nose. As you exhale through the nose, let your breath out very slowly—and with it, relax. Take in another breath and let it out even more slowly. Feel yourself relaxing deeply.*

*Place the awareness of "I" in the center of the heart.*
*Ask yourself: Who am I?*
*Am I the body? The flesh? The bones? The blood? The organs?*
*No, I am not the body!*
*Who am I?*
*Am I the organs of motion?*
*Am I the arms that reach out? No, I am not the arms or the action of reaching.*
*Who am I?*
*Am I the legs that propel the body to move and touch the earth?*
*No, I am not the legs or the movement of the legs.*

*Who am I?*

*Am I the organs of the senses?*

*Am I the eyes that see all sights? No, I am not the eyes or the seeing!*

*Who am I?*

*Am I the ears that hear all sounds? No, I am not the ears or the hearing.*

*Who am I?*

*Am I the nose that smells all scents? No, I am not the nose or the smelling.*

*Who am I?*

*Am I the tongue that tastes and talks? No, I am not the tongue or the sense of taste or the action of speech.*

*Who am I?*

*Am I the skin, the sense of feeling? No, I am not the skin or the sense of touch.*

*Who am I?*

*Observe and experience the following:*

*your eyes and inner and outer seeing*

*your ears and inner and outer hearing*

*your nose and inner and outer smelling*

*your tongue and inner and outer tasting*

*your tongue and inner and outer talking*

*Who am I?*

*Am I the mind?*

*No, I am not the mind.*

*How could I be the mind if I am observing the mind? I must be something other than the mind.*

*Who am I?*

*Am I the emotions?*

*No, I am not the emotions, because I can observe and change the emotions.*

*Who am I?*

*Even the original "I" that was put in the center of the heart is not me. Because I put it there.*

*Who am I?*

*I am beyond all these things. I am absolute truth, absolute knowledge, absolute bliss.*

*Who am I?*

*I am the one who knows.*

# ASTHAANGA YOGA:
## The Eight-Faceted Path

WE FIND THE practical application of Yogic Wisdom distilled into eight dynamic facets. As you were studying the preceding sutras, you might have wondered, "How can *I* possibly realize this?" The answer lies in *Asthaanga Yoga*. It is so often considered the essence that, for many, the whole study of the sutras is termed *Asthaanga Yoga*.

*By embracing* Asthaanga Yoga, *the Eight-Faceted Path,
Intuitive Wisdom dawns and reveals our inner radiance.*

Asthaanga Yoga, the Eight-Faceted Path, embraces:
Yama: *reflection of our true nature*
Niyama: *evolution toward harmony*
Asana: *comfort in being, posture*
Pranayama: *enhancement and guidance of universal* prana
(energy)
Pratyahara: *encouraging the senses to draw within*
Dharana: *gathering and focusing of consciousness inward*
Dhyana: *continuous inward flow of consciousness*
Samadhi: *union with Divine Consciousness*

Yama (*reflection of our true nature*) *is experienced through:*
Ahimsa: *reverence, love, compassion for all*
Satya: *truthfulness, integrity*
Astheya: *generosity, honesty*
Brahmacharya: *balance and moderation of the vital life force*
Aparigraha: *awareness of abundance, fulfillment*

*These great truths are universal and inherent to all beings.*

*If they are altered or ignored, the quality of life is greatly compromised.*

Niyama (*evolution toward harmony*) *encompasses:*
Saucha: *simplicity, purity, refinement*
Santosha: *contentment, being at peace with oneself and others*
Tapas: *igniting the purifying flame*
Swadhaya: *sacred study of the Divine through scripture, nature, and introspection*
Iswara Pranidhana: *wholehearted dedication to the Divine*

*When presented with disquieting thoughts or feelings, cultivate an opposite, elevated attitude. This is* Pratipaksha Bhavana.

*The desire to act upon unwholesome thoughts or actions or to cause or condone others toward these thoughts or actions is preventable. This is also* Pratipaksha Bhavana.

II.28 *By embracing* Asthaanga Yoga, *the Eight-Faceted Path, Intuitive Wisdom dawns and reveals our inner radiance.*

II.29 Asthaanga Yoga, *the Eight-Faceted Path, embraces:*

*Yama:* reflection of our true nature
*Niyama:* evolution toward harmony
*Asana:* comfort in being, posture
*Pranayama:* enhancement and guidance of
    universal *prana* (energy)
*Pratyahara:* encouraging the senses to draw within
*Dharana:* gathering and focusing of consciousness
    inward
*Dhyana:* continuous inward flow of consciousness
*Samadhi:* union with Divine Consciousness

*Asthaanga* is two words. *Astha* means "eight" and *angha* means "intertwining facets." *Angha* is often translated as "limb," and the term can give the impression of a linear ascent, like climbing a tree. Starting at the trunk, we wend our way out to the end of the limb. But instead of a completion, the limbs of this tree end in interconnection. This may be frustrating when we are unable to complete each one in its own turn. But it is an integrated system.

Rather than the image of a single tree or limb, the many facets of *Asthaanga Yoga* are similar to a grove of trees. From the trunk upward, the trees appear to be independent, not connected to one another. However, if we venture several inches below the surface, we will find that these seemingly separate trees have their root systems intertwined. Their interdependency for enduring strength and drawing in of moisture unites them. Each is able to manifest a unique appearance while embracing the same consciousness. Similar to entwined tree roots, we are reminded that *Asthaanga* is not a series of practices to "accomplish"; rather, it is an offering of infinite possibilities and combinations to enhance our way of being. Because of this, we encourage them to interact and function interdependently rather than individually. At times we may choose to single out one or another to help us focus on a particular aspect of our development. After some time, the integration of the other facets will be necessary as we continue our journey inward toward wholeness and discovering our divinity.

Five of these facets are described in the second book, "*Sadhana Pada*: Cultivation of Spiritual Practice." The last three are expounded upon in the third book, "*Vibhuti Pada*: The Divine Manifestation of Power." This structure is meant to suggest that *Dharana* (contemplation), *Dhyana* (meditation), and *Samadhi* (union with Divine Consciousness) are not practices in themselves but states that blossom through the nurturing practices that preceded them.

Through the process of incarnation, our finite bodies must accommodate the vast and infinite ocean of consciousness, as it infuses divine qualities into our human life. As human beings, we hope to reflect the higher states of consciousness along with our humanity. The Eight-Faceted Path encourages that integration.

**Asthaanga Yoga *is the Eight-Faceted Path*.**


## II.30 Yama *(reflection of our true nature) is experienced through:*

> *Ahimsa:* reverence, love, compassion for all
> *Satya:* truthfulness, integrity

*Astheya:* generosity, honesty
*Brahmacharya:* balance and moderation of the vital
   life force
*Aparigraha:* awareness of abundance, fulfillment

## THE TWO PINNACLES OF DYNAMIC ENERGY

*Yama* (reflection of our true nature) and *Niyama* (evolution toward harmony) are the first two facets of *Asthaanga*.

Within each of the two facets *Yama* and *Niyama,* there are five additional facets encouraging us to live in peace, honoring the spirit at each moment. Imagine two round brilliant-cut diamonds meshed together at the top, each directing energy to or from the pinnacle. The pinnacles represent the foremost qualities of each: *Ahimsa* in *Yama* and *Iswara Pranidhana* in *Niyama.* When we revere all as ourselves through *Ahimsa,* the other four qualities of *Yama—Satya,* (truthfulness), *Astheya* (generosity), *Brahmacharya* (moderation), and *Aparigraha* (abundance)—are naturally present.

*Iswara Pranidhana,* wholehearted dedication to the Divine, conveys the essence of the four other *Niyamas: Saucha* (simplicity), *Santosha* (contentment), *Tapas* (igniting the purifying flame), and *Swadhaya* (sacred study). The integration of the *Yamas* and *Niyamas* in our lives reflects the beauty and light of a diamond. Everything that is touched by these will then reproduce its own beauty and light.

## INSPIRED OFFERINGS, NOT COMMANDMENTS

Often, to simplify the enormous breadth and depth of the *Yamas* and *Niyamas,* they are called the "do's and don'ts of Yoga" or sometimes the "ten commandments of Yoga." This is taking a highly refined and virtuous way of living, expressed throughout the millennia, and reducing it to a finger-wagging image: "If you do not do this or that, you will be punished." When observed on a subtler level, the *Yamas* and *Niyamas* seem to be more of a tribute to being, affirming our already divine nature.

During the time period when the Ten Commandments were delivered, the Divine was represented as a strong and very strict patriarch. The people's morals and attitudes had diminished, and many thought that drastic measures were needed to facilitate a change.

During the time when the ideals of the *Yamas* and *Niyamas* were formulated, the atmosphere was of a different nature. It was during the Golden Age (*Sat Yuga*), and virtue still reigned. Nonetheless, the steady decline in consciousness was evident. Everyone was eager to find a way to preserve these values. The positive way people lived their lives was reflected in their wisdom.

**Yama:** *reflection of our true nature.*

It is up to each of us in our hearts to decide which level of consciousness we want to abide in, in our spiritual life and in the world. As you read and practice the *Yamas* and *Niyamas,* feel that they are sparking your Golden Age (*Sat Yuga*) consciousness, where virtue is supreme. These two giant pyramids of virtue are given to us so that we may remember to live our lives in a noble and sacred way.

Knowing the importance of repeating a statement in the affirmative, I have chosen to translate (as much as I possibly could) using positive, life-affirming language. If we say, "I will *not* eat sugar today," the human mind sees through the "not" and concentrates on the sugar. In the same way, continually reading translations formed in the negative evokes Iron Age (*Kali Yuga*) consciousness, rather than our natural effulgence shining through from the Golden Age (*Sat Yuga*).

When an athlete is in training, positive phrasing is found to be most effective. "Don't put your elbows out when you swing that golf club" may actually cause the undesirable effect. Instead, "Keep your elbows in when you swing" is found to elicit better results.

When words or phrases evoke fear, punishment, or denial of pleasure, they encroach on our spiritual practices and diminish rather than enhance the glory of our true nature. By embracing everything as divine, our all-loving nature is radiantly revealed.

Bring forth the Golden Age (*Sat Yuga*) consciousness within the Iron Age (*Kali Yuga*) by upholding these divine qualities. Be open-hearted as the facets of *Asthaanga Yoga* unfurl the realization of your true nature.

Yama: *reflection of our true nature.*

II.31 *These great truths are universal and inherent to all beings. If they are altered or ignored, the quality of life is greatly compromised.*

We can all make excuses and find reasons for not upholding these declarations, even when our quality of life is affected. The infractions may seem so *minor* that they remain unnoticed; yet some part of us is deeply affected. In those quiet moments by ourselves, we find the incongruities between who we are and who we think we are emerging. They tend to be so subtle that although we may be aware that something is bothering us, we are unable to discern its origin. If something is said that inadvertently awakens those opposing thoughts and feelings, we may overreact without understanding the real cause of the distress.

One of the most important ways to keep our intention is the power of *satsang* (company of those who share the same truth).

When we need reassurance to stay focused on the practices, whom do we call on? If it is someone who already has experienced the benefits of practice, we will receive encouragement to continue. Without the same understanding, a well-meaning friend might convince us to venture onward to other horizons.

*The Yama and Niyama are expressed in all aspects of our thoughts, words, and actions.* This is what allows them to be at the same time powerful and challenging to abide by.

*These great truths are universal and inherent to all beings. If they are altered or ignored, the quality of life is greatly compromised.*

## II.32 Niyama *(evolution toward harmony)* encompasses:

*Saucha:* simplicity, purity, refinement
*Santosha:* contentment, being at peace with oneself and others
*Tapas:* igniting the purifying flame
*Swadhaya:* sacred study of the Divine through scripture, nature, and introspection
*Iswara Pranidhana:* wholehearted dedication to the Divine

Here *Iswara Pranidhana* is at the pinnacle of the diamond pyramid. All of the *Niyamas* are enhanced when *Iswara Pranidhana* is honored, and it is honored when we live in harmony with the other four *Niyamas*.

**Niyama:** *evolution toward harmony.*

## II.33 *When presented with disquieting thoughts or feelings, cultivate an opposite, elevated attitude. This is* Pratipaksha Bhavana.

This is one of my favorite sutras because it helps to change *my* attitude rather than hoping to change the situation or the people who "cause me" to be unhappy. It is a key practice that enables us to remain in harmony, balanced, and openhearted.

*Pratipaksha* offers the option of cultivating the opposite thoughts, feelings, and actions. *Bhavana* is the Sanskrit root of our English verb "to be." Together they encourage us to reverse our attitude, to embrace a noble way of being.

Daily life presents us with a plethora of frustrations and challenges. Our hope is that as our consciousness blossoms, life's trials will ease. It is not always the case; often the situations that were previously endured gracefully affect us *more*. With clarity we realize that changing the situation may not be possible; rather, we see that changing our attitude allows peace to bloom.

We may stubbornly hold the belief that others cause our problems and inconveniences. In those situations we may appoint ourselves as their teachers to show them the correct way to act. From that attitude our egos enlarge, leaving us with less room for insight. If you routinely feel it is the other person's fault, take another look, this time from a different perspective.

*When presented with disquieting thoughts or feelings, cultivate an opposite, elevated attitude. This is* **Pratipaksha Bhavana.**

*Pratipaksha Bhavana* is a simple and direct way of keeping our minds calm and our hearts open. How often during the day do unwanted thoughts or feelings pop up to disturb your calm? Some days there might be too many to count!

When we are aware of these unfavorable attitudes *before* they manifest as word or action, we retain the power to reverse them. Do you feel fear? Cultivate courage. Anger? Cultivate love. Try substituting not just a word but a whole scene or action. Perhaps you are in the midst of a heated discussion with your spouse when, from another room, you hear your sweet baby cooing. Chances are as soon as you hear the first sound, your mind and heart will leave the disagreement, and your anger will melt away as your heart opens to your child. The next time you feel annoyed with anyone, invoke an image like the face of your sweet baby, or perhaps a budding flower or a brilliant sunset. The person worthy of your discontent may suddenly appear more vulnerable as you feel more loving. The best part is that you both reap the benefits.

## MAKE A DIFFICULT PERSON YOUR PERSONAL DEITY

There was a time while living at the ashram that I was in charge of a large department with many ashramites to supervise. One quite grumpy monk very much resented doing anything that was asked of him, especially if a woman issued the directive. Each morning, I dreaded telling him the needs of the day. He remained quiet as he stood in front of me, but as he turned and walked away he would mutter unkind words. It very much disturbed me, but no amount of words or gestures could soothe him.

Calling on *Pratipaksha Bhavana,* I designed a spiritual practice in which he was the principal deity. Each day as he entered my office, I would imagine placing a garland of flowers over his head and touching his feet. As he turned to walk away, murmuring under his breath, my hands joined together in a *pranam* to wish him well. This "worship" continued and initiated itself each time he passed by. The practice then sprang into being each time I thought about him. Of course, no one else knew about it; only my mind and heart held the secret.

One week into the practice, I was no longer stifling a visceral reaction to run when I saw him. The practice was benefiting me in many ways. My mind and heart were now focusing on flower garlands and worship rather than dwelling on a strategy to avoid grumpy people.

One morning, at the usual time, he appeared in my office and, with a surprised tone, said, "You know that I do not like you very much, don't you?" I only nodded "yes," so as to not give my voice a chance to betray me. "Well, it's a funny thing," he continued, "but in the last week, I find that I am actually starting to look forward to seeing you, well, just a little bit. I can't figure out why. Do you know?"

Smiling on the inside, I said, "Well, perhaps we are both changing and our reason for disliking each other is fading away." I kept up the practice for months. I cannot say we became best friends, but we both were able to say, "We like each other."

**When presented with disquieting thoughts or feelings, cultivate an opposite, elevated attitude. This is Pratipaksha Bhavana.**

## EXPERIENCING THE PROFOUND EFFECT OF CHANGING YOUR ATTITUDE

*Sit comfortably.*

*Think of a quality that you would like to invite into your life. A simple one- or two-word phrase is best. It could be "peace," "joy," "cooperation," "adaptability," etc. (For this example we will use "joy.")*

*Bring forth an aspect of yourself that no longer fosters the person you want to be. Can you tell where in your body it is stored? If possible, put a name to it—"self-righteousness," "stubbornness," "anger," etc. (For this example we will use "resentment.")*

*Now choose a quality that you would like to send out to the world. It could be the same or a different one than you chose to bring into your life. (For this example we will use the quality of "peace.")*

*Begin to take in and release deep, full breaths.*

*As you breathe in, allow the mind and heart to integrate the quality of joy into your being. Feel joy infusing each cell, encircling the place where you are holding resentment, and allow the unwanted feeling to dissipate.*

*As you breathe out, let joy transform resentment into peace and send it as your wish for the world.*

*(When the mind is focused as in this practice, it is important not to hold the breath or breathe out the negative emotion. Through the breath the mind gains power, and with focus the negative is exaggerated rather than calmed. It is fun to watch the resentment dissolve and transform into peace!)*

## EXPERIENCING THE EFFECTS THIS HAS ON DIFFICULT PEOPLE AND SITUATIONS

*As you feel comfortable with the previous practice, use it in a variety of situations with people or things that cause you to become annoyed.*

*Begin to breathe in a positive quality (it could be the same or different than the one you used in the last practice); as you breathe out, send a directed wish to them.*

*To add to the power, notice something you like about that person. That alone is enough to change your vibrational quality. (The thing you like about the person might be as simple as a pretty blouse or the color of a necktie.)*

*Continue the imagery until the negative feelings subside or you are able to remove yourself from the circumstances. If it is a situation you frequently encounter, repeat this practice as often as possible and be amazed at the change in both you and them.*

II.34 *The desire to act upon unwholesome thoughts or actions or to cause or condone others toward these thoughts or actions is preventable. This is also* Pratipaksha Bhavana.

Even the *desire* to do something hurtful to another can be pacified by *Pratipaksha Bhavana.* This also encompasses the impulse to stand by and allow hurtful actions to happen to others. There are situations in which we may feel helpless given the actions being taken by either an individual or a government. Sometimes our only recourse is to peacefully protest, petition, write letters, or speak out in some way. Through this we may assuage our exasperation and hope that our intervention will elicit some benefit.

It seems like many years ago that I discovered that the simple act of eating a grape was contributing to the suffering of many.

Learning of the grape pickers' plight, many of us joined together in a boycott, our hearts leaping in solidarity. Even now, a long time hence, this self-imposed act of camaraderie makes me hesitate when popping a tasty grape in my mouth.

We hear much about companies using child labor or abusing workers. Taking action even in the smallest way (such as not buying the product) allows the mind and the heart to know they are contributing to the solution, not the problem.

It is important for retaining our peace that the protests, boycotts, letters, and petitions be arranged in a calm nature. Otherwise, we unknowingly contribute to the injury. When participating in a peace demonstration, remember to bring your peace with you and keep it strong. It is from this cocoon of peace that the power emerges.

*The desire to act upon unwholesome thoughts or actions or to cause or condone others toward these thoughts or actions is preventable. This is also* **Pratipaksha Bhavana.**

# YAMA:
## Reflection of Our True Nature

HERE WE EXPLORE FIVE inner facets of *Asthaanga Yoga* called *Yama*. They encourage us to live in peace with ourselves and one another.

*Embracing reverence and love for all (Ahimsa), we experience oneness.*

*Dedicated to truth and integrity (Satya), our thoughts, words, and actions gain the power to manifest.*

*Abiding in generosity and honesty (Astheya), material and spiritual prosperity is bestowed.*

*Devoted to living a balanced and moderate life (Brahmacharya), the scope of one's life force becomes boundless.*

*Acknowledging abundance (Aparigraha), we recognize the blessings in everything and gain insights into the purpose of our worldly existence.*

## II.35 *Embracing reverence and love for all* (Ahimsa), *we experience oneness.*

*Ahimsa,* the pinnacle of the diamond pyramid, gives brilliance to the *Yamas.* Sanctifying every moment of the day with reverence and love, the other four *Yamas* easily integrate into our lives.

The practice of *Ahimsa* transports us to Golden Age (*Sat Yuga*) awareness, where the entire world of people, animals, plants, and in-animate objects is our family and friends, and ultimately we are one.

> To those that lowly creep, I am the self in all.
>
> —Swami Vivekananda

As babies, we see the world through pure hearts and open eyes. We live the purity of *Ahimsa,* experiencing oneness with every-one and everything. With the development of the mind's ability to discriminate, differences emerge. We must then be constantly reminded that even though people and things appear to be differ-ent, in our essence we are all the same.

Throughout time, many religious stories and books underplayed the loving and compassionate aspect of the Divine, accentuating instead the fearful and punitive roles. Fear, rationalized the story-tellers, would have the power to make us humble and thus believe in virtuous rules.

## THE MASCULINE AND FEMININE QUALITIES IN THE SACRED TEXTS

The (masculine) qualities of fury and punishment in the Old and New Testaments cry out for balance. Clandestinely woven through-out the Hebrew Bible is the term *rachamim,* the feminine quality of mercy and compassion that is attributed to God's softer side. Its meaning is derived from *rechem,* meaning maternal or womb-like attributes. *Rachamim* perpetuates the dynamic regenerative power millions have felt from this great scripture for thousands of years. With the translation into modern languages, the representation and wording of the feminine are obscured, and the masculine qualities are brought front and center. It is important to remember that all life is a balance, and a delicate one at that.

The New Testament has the benefit of the great parables of Jesus's compassion. Throughout the scripture, he is constantly coming to the defense of the wrongly accused and the outcasts of society, showing us that we are all the same in our hearts. Depending upon who is narrating, the compassion is underscored or overlooked. The appearances and visitations of Mother Mary to small clusters of openhearted devotees (as narrated through *their* devoted memoirs) allow her to bestow limitless compassion to the multitudes.

In the Bhagavad Gita, Sri Krishna plays both the strict teacher and the loving, compassionate friend. The story vacillates between the harshness of fighting a righteous war and the peace of recognizing the Divine in all. It is up to the reader to choose to fight or nestle into the compassion Lord Krishna has for all his devotees.

Many examples from the holy scriptures tantalize us with the kind of power that comes from exerting our might and overcoming fear. Less often we are reminded that abounding in love and compassion, we are led to revere, not fear, the Divine.

Mahatma Gandhi employed the principles of *Ahimsa,* which he so dearly cherished, in dealing with the foreign intruders ruling India. He inspired all the citizens of India to love their enemy. The foreign empire, confused by the unforeseen attitude, was brought to its knees. The British retreated in peace, holding Mahatma Gandhi in the highest esteem. By encasing the principles of *Ahimsa* in his heart, he dearly respected even those who caused him harm.

Gandhi remains a great inspiration, exemplifying compassion in the face of adversity.

> Service is not possible unless it is rooted in love and compassion. The best way to find yourself is to lose yourself in the service of others.
>
> —*Mahatma Gandhi*

*Embracing reverence and love for all* (Ahimsa), *we experience oneness.*

Most often this exalted virtue of *Ahimsa* is translated simply as "nonharming" or even "nonviolence." Again we visit the idea of placing a "non" in front of a negative trait, telling us what *not to do* instead of how to espouse our true nature. It implies that we are "inherently" violent and that mischief may be lurking somewhere in the background of our minds. (Often *Yama* is translated as "restraints.") You may even be insulted by the accusation, protesting, "I do not *harm* anyone. I am not *violent*. This sutra is not meant for me!" Neither violence nor harming was implied in the Golden Age (*Sat Yuga*), only reverence and compassion. This is where we discover the vast chasm between *not killing* or *not doing harm* and embracing reverence and love. *Ahimsa* in the latter implies that our nature is to be compassionate, and when we practice *Ahimsa* fully, all living things that come into our presence experience it.

"My religion is kindness," humbly says His Holiness the Dalai Lama, a distinguished living example of *Ahimsa*.

Embracing the great virtue of *Ahimsa* brings the knowledge that each of us feels pain, joy, disappointment, love—the full spectrum of emotions. We develop an empathy with others and our individual experience becomes the experience of all.

As we open our hearts, *Ahimsa* elegantly beams reverence and love to the many facets of our life. We accept the importance of respecting all, even those who threaten or harm us physically or emotionally. Yet the part that many of us forget is *to treat ourselves with that same reverence and love.*

The Bible compassionately tells us to "love thy neighbor as thyself." The difficult lesson for many of us is to learn to love and serve ourselves first.

*Embracing reverence and love for all* (Ahimsa), *we experience oneness.*

When we refuse to take the time to treat our bodies, emotions, and minds with reverence and love, they will often remind us—not so kindly—by failing to respond when we need them. Our ability to think clearly recedes. We may experience sadness or depression. After a time our lack of ease may allow disease to creep into our life. Then we are obliged to take time for ourselves. It is much more pleasant and fun to do it willingly, before any dis-ease invites itself to your life. Love for oneself is love for all.

Listen to the wisdom of your own physical heart. A mighty pump, it selflessly distributes blood throughout the body during your entire life. The heart itself first consumes the fresh oxygenated blood coming from the lungs. The heart is intuitive enough to know that it must take care of itself so it has the fortitude to then pump the blood out to oxygenate the rest of the body. It doesn't say, "Oh, the stomach seems to need the blood because it is digesting right now. I'll send it there first."

Remembering this simple illustration from the heart, we learn that in order to better serve others, we must provide for ourselves first. It is only then that we are inspired to live for the good of all.

For most of us the practice of *Ahimsa* is shown in thousands of small actions and words throughout the day. In other countries, it inspires me to observe flower garlands adorning trucks, cars, and tractors while prized cows, goats, bulls, and camels are honored with gaily colored decorations. In this way everything is beautiful and respected. We often forget that consciousness resides in every molecule, that what we put forth reflects back to us.

*Embracing reverence and love for all* (Ahimsa), *we experience oneness.*

## EVEN A CAR HAS CONSCIOUSNESS

One time when I was traveling with Sri Swami Satchidanandaji, we were late for a *satsang* (spiritual gathering). After hastily opening the car door for him, Susan noisily slammed the door shut. Immediately, Sri Swamiji turned around and, with a look of alarm, asked her to apologize to the car. Feeling ridiculous and hoping that he was joking, she continued to walk. Sri Swamiji said, "Don't you realize what service this car has done for us? Without its assistance we would not be able to come this distance. It has brought us here safely and in comfort. For that service you, thoughtlessly, have slammed its door and caused the whole car to vibrate and be hurt." After that heartfelt explanation, Susan walked back to the car and, with a gentle caress, explained how sorry she was to have slammed the door. The cars I drive, even today, still benefit from this great lesson of long ago.

Even if you inadvertently harm yourself or others, generously bathe the injury in love and compassion. *Ahimsa* is a permanent reminder for those of us determined to live each moment with the knowledge that we are all divine.

> If you truly loved yourself, you could never hurt another.
> —*Lord Buddha*

*Embracing reverence and love for all* (Ahimsa), *we experience oneness.*

## EXPERIENCING THE JOY OF LIVING WITH REVERENCE FOR ALL (*AHIMSA*)

Ahimsa *is a vast and continuous practice. Rather than waking up tomorrow morning and vowing to have reverence for everyone and everything all the time, it is better to choose something specific and obvious. Giving yourself the opportunity to succeed is in itself* Ahimsa.

*Is there a person or a situation that could assist you in your practice? Is there someone whom you have treated unkindly or who has treated you unkindly? Perhaps it was someone at the office who could be soothed by an offering of flowers or a healthy treat. Healing the hurt that already exists is a great beginning to the practice of* Ahimsa.

## EXPERIENCING HAVING REVERENCE FOR THE SMALL AND SIMPLE ASPECTS OF LIFE

*For continuous remembrance of* Ahimsa, *try embracing the simple.*

*Each time you close a drawer or a door, do so with gentleness and reverence, affirming that it, too, has consciousness. Each day we close scores of drawers and doors, helping to bring* Ahimsa *into the moment.*

*Begin to observe the way you walk. Is your step light or heavy? Do you clunk around the house or office? Sometimes the smallest and lightest people make the loudest noises. It is not physical size; it is mental consciousness. Are you considerate of others on floors below you? Are your shoes leaving scuff marks on the floor?*

*When you walk outside on the grass, are you aware of all the little creatures that live in that same earth? Awareness blesses them as your foot steps softly.*

*Add other practices as your consciousness flourishes. Always keep* Ahimsa *at the center of your thoughts, words, and actions.*

## II.36 *Dedicated to truth and integrity* (Satya), *our thoughts, words, and actions gain the power to manifest.*

*Satya* is a profound virtue espoused by most major traditions as a dedication to the unspoken truth that nestles in our hearts. Through *Satya* we embrace the depth of truth that words can only hope to convey.

There are many ways to access the truth. The depth of our heart's chasm measures the integrity necessary to approach real truth. The power (Shakti) of truth is created through the alchemy of personal integrity, knowledge, and humility.

Can you "feel" truth as a physical reaction to the energy that is present, long before the mind has captured the words? Tears may fall spontaneously as your heart unfolds, ready to receive. With energy and words that dim truth, do you experience a tightening in the body that releases a wash of fear and anxiety? The heart rests when it is in *Satya*.

> Is it true? Is it kind? Is it necessary?
>
> —*Sufi saying*

Our words are so very powerful that we often do not realize the benefits or consequences they bestow on others or ourselves. Although our actions may appear to be benevolent, our words or thoughts may betray us with their expressions. Sometimes we misunderstand the true purpose of *Satya*.

## TRUTH OR OPINION?

Walking down the street in Manhattan, I overheard a conversation. "It's too bad if she is angry with me," a woman said with indignation.

"You were very harsh with her," replied her kind companion.

"I was just telling her *the truth*! She can't blame her hurt feelings on me!"

"Maybe what you expressed was not the truth but *your interpretation* of the truth," her friend softly offered.

A conversation similar to this one takes place countless times a day. Often we mistake the prejudices that are formed through the colored lenses of our minds for the truth. Our words are then formed based on this formula. When our minds and hearts remain expanded, truth shines through.

As we learn to live in *Satya*, we become familiar with where integrity and truth lie. As we step into that stream, all our experiences are invited to flow along in the same direction. The more we live not just *our* version of the truth but the truth itself, the more the other aspects of our life neatly join the order.

***Dedicated to truth and integrity* (Satya)*, our thoughts, words, and actions gain the power to manifest.***

> A word is a bird and the teeth are the cage; if we let the bird fly,
> we can never get it back.
>
> —*Sri Swami Sivananadaji*

Getting ready to go out, your friend comes out of the bathroom and asks, "How do you like my new dress?" Withholding an audible gasp, you pause for a second. What was she thinking to buy a dress like that? Both the color and the style are awful. She will be stared at and laughed at if she goes to the party like that. What to do? If you tell her that you dislike the dress, you will ruin her evening. If you don't tell her how you feel, you are not living in integrity with your heart. Not a simple choice.

Take a moment to breathe deeply. As you do, remember that there were many people who thought this dress was beautiful. There was the one who designed it, the one who sewed it, the buyer at the store, and, lastly, your dear friend. Maybe, just maybe, it is your *opinion* of the dress, not the absolute truth.

"*You* look beautiful tonight, radiant as always." The decision to tell her your version of the truth tomorrow rather than tonight saves a great deal of hurt feelings.

> I've learned that people will forget what you said, people will forget what you did, but people will never forget how you made them feel.
>
> —*Maya Angelou*

Can you remember a time when you attempted to cover up a falsehood? Did it seem as though the whole world was there to expose you? At other times, when in alignment with your integrity, the potency of the truth could be felt everywhere you went.

## GOSSIPING DEFUSES OUR NERVOUS SYSTEMS

The so-called fight-or-flight syndrome is considered a normal male response to a sympathetic nervous system reaction. The response is different when the same feelings are elicited in a woman's nervous system. As women, we process our stress differently from men. If there is great danger, a man's natural instinct is either to fight or to flee.

Being maternal by nature, women are engineered to protect. When danger approaches, we become quiet and still and ask our children to respond the same way. What then happens when the danger passes? We must somehow allow that internalized fear to dissipate. Men can release stress by working it out in the gym. While women receive *some* benefit from a physical release, we often find more comfort in sharing and expressing feelings with others. If this is not done, our feelings burrow deep within; sadly, this normal instinct to freeze and withdraw often leads us to depression. A woman's more verbal response to emotionally charged events has been misunderstood and criticized for ages.

The now-derogatory term "gossip" originally meant "to see God" or "godparent." Gossiping actually started as an alarm system. Women hanging clothes to dry would pass on news of the town, warnings, or any unpleasant experiences, especially with abusive men. They would whisper these messages hoping to protect others from this peril. When the men found out that their names were being dragged through the mud (or in this case the clean sheets), they decreed a severe punishment for any gossiping.

> We are not afraid to follow truth wherever it may lead.
>
> —*Thomas Jefferson*

> If in doubt whether to observe *Ahimsa* or *Satya,* always go with *Ahimsa.*
>
> —*Swami Vivekananda*

*Dedicated to truth and integrity (Satya), our thoughts, words, and actions gain the power to manifest.*

## EXPERIENCING TRUTH AND INTEGRITY (*SATYA*)

*Can you "feel" truth? How does it affect you when you read or hear something that you know to be true? Untrue?*

*Observe where on your body you feel truth and untruth.*

*To further enhance this practice of observation, choose an idea or a concept that you "feel" is untrue. Where is that conviction coming from? Did you ever believe it to be true?*

*Choose a concept that you feel is true. Where is that conviction coming from? Did you ever have any doubt?*

*Can you feel both truth and untruth reverberate in your body, thoughts, and feelings?*

*How do they then manifest in your speech and action?*

*How do they manifest in your life?*

*Do you find your integrity compromised or enhanced?*

*Gradually begin to trust and accept your inner knowing.*

*There is much in this world that will support you when you have a deep inner conviction.*

## II.37 *Abiding in generosity and honesty* (Astheya), *material and spiritual prosperity is bestowed.*

Our world encourages us to achieve more, amass more, and yet most of us feel we are lacking in many aspects of our life. *Astheya* has the power to initiate us into material and spiritual prosperity beyond our greatest expectations.

On a philosophical level we understand that we came into this world free of material possessions and when we leave, we leave with nothing. Even our bodies that were provided for us must stay, affirming that what we use on this earth belongs to the earth. Casually we speak about owning land or a house, yet can we move that acre of land from Montana to Florida in the winter months for warmth? It seems more like the earth is housing *us*, owning *us*.

Knowing all this, we still think of things as "mine." We attach strong possessive pronouns before objects, as if that protected us from their ever leaving us: *my* house, *her* car, *his* pen. We then become offended if someone takes something that is *mine*. We legislate to protect ourselves from thieves, but the laws are not able to protect us from the *fear* of loss. When we don the attitude of caretakers instead of owners, we enjoy things when they come and let them go with ease. It is nature's rhythm: All things come *and* all things go.

## GIVING PERMISSION TO GIVE

One of my sister monks was enjoying the water cascading down her back when she realized she had forgotten to bring her shampoo into the shower. Not wanting to stop, dry off, or drip water onto the floor, she pondered using *my* shampoo, which was sitting on the shelf. After silently asking my permission, she proceeded to lather up. At the same moment the image of her using my shampoo came to me. Immediately, permission was joyfully granted.

"You are always welcome to use my shampoo," I greeted her as she walked from the shower room wrapped in a towel. "How did you know?" she asked. I answered, "I felt your 'call for permission' and it was instantly given."

> If someone asks for your shirt, give them your coat also.
>
> —*New Testament*

*Abiding in generosity and honesty* (Astheya), *material and spiritual prosperity is bestowed.*

## GIVING GENEROUSLY OF ONESELF

*Astheya* encompasses not only generosity with money and giving of things, but also generosity with time and giving from our hearts. When you set a time for an appointment, make it a priority to be there *on time*. Otherwise you are taking energy from the person you are scheduled to meet. Your intentions may be honorable as you set your departure time, but there are always one or two quick things you could do before leaving. "Oh, well, I might be *slightly* late, but that's okay," you think to yourself. That kind of thinking leads us away from an openhearted exchange. When we do meet, the beginning of the interaction is likely to be very uncomfortable. You will feel the need to apologize or explain. She will have arranged her schedule to fit this allotted time, perhaps, making sacrifices so she could be on time. When she waits for you, you become a thief, stealing her time. If this becomes a frequent occurrence, even longtime friendships can be strained. Much of the spiritual energy that you are accruing will dissipate.

Ever have the experience of reading an interesting email when you are interrupted by a phone call from a distressed friend? Are you able to draw your mind from the email and generously give her your full heart and mind? Or do you let her talk as you continue to be involved with the email? Generosity gives great gifts in many small ways.

In the face of great tragedy, people are known to open their hearts to those considered strangers just minutes before. Others needing an outlet for their pain and frustration may intentionally snatch any remnants of calm they feel from others.

After the catastrophic events of September 11, 2001, the devastation continued as many sought to blame and punish the perpetrators of this heinous crime. In lieu of a healthy outlet, their frustrations continued to be fueled by the inability to locate the offenders. Feelings of helplessness stoked the rage as it burst out, scorching an innocent population. The wave of hatred overtook and stole what little safety was left in many ethnic communities guilty of nothing more than having the same religious background or national origin as the terrorists.

For most parents the original disaster was difficult enough to explain to their children. They were now grasping for whatever goodness they could gather to protect the innocence of their children and to calm the colossal fear. Humbly they sought the sage advice of one of the icons of kindheartedness in the world of children. Mr. Rogers, a longtime TV host and minister, encouraged and empowered countless children to live with kindness and love. His advice whispers the secret of generosity from time immemorial: "Tell the children to watch the helpers. Their generosity of heart and time is an inspiration to us all. It can help soothe our pain as it encourages our hearts to open."

*Abiding in generosity and honesty* (Astheya)*, material and spiritual prosperity is bestowed.*

The vibration of *Astheya* magnifies our experience of prosperity, smoothing the way for us to give generously to others. At times when our hearts are open, generosity cascades unencumbered. At other times, we must recall when we were bathed in our own generosity or that of another, and how blessed we felt.

In our lives we have many occasions to give. In the simplest way, *Astheya* tells us not to steal. As it expands your heart, it says, *give*. For maximum benefit, do not even wait for someone to ask; be alert, and never miss an opportunity to give, give, give. Sri Swami Sivananadaji's students who hoped to emulate his most generous nature gave him the nickname "Swami Give-*ananda*" (the bliss of giving).

> To believe in something, and not to live it, is dishonest.
>
> —*Mahatma Gandhi*

**Abiding in generosity and honesty** (Astheya), **material and spiritual prosperity is bestowed.**

## EXPERIENCING THE GRACE OF GENEROSITY AND HONESTY (*ASTHEYA*)

*Observe your life, and with a generous heart envision the great and small ways you experience wealth and prosperity. Make a list. The list may include the bounty of food you have access to whenever you feel hunger, or your closet filled with clothes for all types of weather and conditions and events.*

*Notice if your comfort expands to giving generously to others. Or do you still feel you need more before you can do that?*

*From the material, move toward generosity of time. Are you al-*
*ways ready to greet others and be helpful? Do you keep others*
*waiting? Can you stop what you are doing to respect the other*
*person's schedule?*

*Observe the way your heart can be generous in giving service to*
*others.*

*In what ways are you generous with yourself? Do you take the*
*time to nurture yourself on all levels?*

*In what small ways can you expand your generosity on a daily*
*basis? As your generosity expands, your heart's capacity to give*
*will increase incrementally.*

## II.38 *Devoted to living a balanced and moderate life* (Brahmacharya), *the scope of one's life force becomes boundless.*

Our journey through the *Yamas* is reminding us to blend our human and divine natures by reflecting reverence for all (*Ahimsa*) and living in truth (*Satya*) and generosity (*Astheya*). We are now introduced to the concept of moderation and balance, *Brahmacharya*. Through this practice we are able to orchestrate the glorious dance between our divine nature and human nature. Each is fueled by the vital energy that is generated as we emulate, rather than resist, nature's beautiful patterns.

## DON'T UPSET MOTHER NATURE!

When nature's balance is upset and large amounts of energy are deployed at one time, the repercussions can be devastating. A raging forest fire, a hurricane, a blizzard, a volcanic eruption, an earthquake: All are dynamic yet destructive releases of nature's power. Fortunately, these flare-ups are infrequent, and most of the time we enjoy nature's changes with metronome-like regularity, such as night and day, summer and winter, sun and rain.

Our bodies, minds, and emotions also respond positively to regular cycles and schedules. If we are fortunate, balance and moderation frame our lives, and very little of our vital energy is spent making adjustments or restoring equilibrium.

*Brahmacharya,* the art of living a moderate life, is a challenging practice in our modern society. When times were simpler, we were more aware and respectful of our bodies, minds, and emotions. The need to adjust our energy was heeded before our energy was depleted ("before" is key). A farmer, knowingly or unknowingly, designs her or his lifestyle according to the fluctuations of nature's cycles. During the planting and harvest time, she or he understands that a large outpouring of energy is necessary. The respite needed to replenish the weary body will come naturally with the shorter days and longer nights of winter. The rhythm of the seasons *naturally* restores balance.

In these modern times, because of great technological advances, our activities no longer depend on times of day or the seasons. We have the ability to control heat and cold, light and darkness. Manipulating nature in this way seems to encourage everything *but* moderation. The concept of moderation is usurped by the "do more and then do much more" attitude. If our tendency is toward overactivity, society waves our speeding train onward. Earning an income while living a life of balance seems more difficult in these contemporary times.

## RESPECTING OUR VITAL ENERGY

Relating to vital energy is similar to the way we relate to our monetary energy. If I have one hundred dollars in my bank account, then
that is the most I should spend. If I spent the entire hundred dollars, then I would technically not have any more money to spend.
However, if I decided to spend one hundred dollars and borrow
another fifty dollars, I would not just be depleted; I would now be
in debt. If this continued, I might borrow more to pay off the loan
and go deeper into debt. With this large depletion, how would it be
possible to generate *more* to pay back what I owed?

Translating this way of thinking back to our own personal energy, if we live in moderation, we have plenty of energy to spend.
We can spend it in many ways. Some can go into service, some
for fun and pleasure, and there will still be plenty available for our
spiritual practices. If we overspend our portion of energy and go
into debt, the vitality and vigor needed for spiritual practice will
be unavailable.

We all know the feeling after eating a big holiday dinner. Our
belly is so stuffed full of food that we are able only to lie on the
couch, groaning. Even for the next few days, we will feel exhausted
and lethargic, having overdrawn our energy account trying to digest
and assimilate the enormous quantity of food. Experiencing this
discomfort, we then tend to swing to the other extreme and eat too
little. This depletes the vitality and strength needed to nourish the
mind, emotions, and body. Only when the physical realm is in a
state of balance is there ample energy to drive us to the more subtle
spiritual vistas.

Overeating is only *one* of the ways we expend this energy. All of
our senses can be enablers. Too much TV, computer work, even
reading will draw on and deplete our vital force. Extreme physical
exercise may leave us feeling exhausted. Too-frequent sexual activity without emotional content causes depletion. Listening to very

loud music or talking too much both create an energetic liability. For our life force to remain strong and available, *all* aspects of our lives need to be balanced.

> Yoga is not for one who eats too much, or for one who fasts too much, nor sleeps too much or sleeps too little, but instead lives in a harmonious flow along the middle path.
>
> —Bhagavad Gita

*Devoted to living a balanced and moderate life* (**Brahmacharya**), *the scope of one's life force becomes boundless.*

## THE POWER OF SEXUAL ENERGY

If *Brahmacharya* is meant to convey a sense of balance and moderation in our life, why is it usually translated as "celibacy" or "continence"? About the time the sutras and other holy books of India were being translated into English, much of Western Europe was enmeshed in a puritanical mindset. This influenced their interpretation of the Bible, which then manipulated their outlook on life.

This mindset brought with it explicit doctrine prohibiting any sexual expression in thought, word, or action. (It was allowed only for procreation, and no one had better enjoy it!) Repressing sexual expression caused monumental adverse effects both on physical health and on emotional stability. The women became the evil courtesans enticing innocent men to act against God. Remember, this was the time when women were persecuted for being women! Even with all the guilt and apprehension, the human species continued to reproduce, unconcerned about fundamentalist doctrine. The Western religious fundamentalists living in India felt it their hallowed duty to impose the same puritanical values on their hosts' way of life. The restrictions were reflected in both the secular and religious realms.

## WOMAN AS TEMPTRESS

Of course the *women* of India were targeted, and a decree to alter their way of dressing was issued. For thousands of years, the traditional dress was a sari. Many yards of unsewn fabric were wound around the waist, covering the lower part of the body, and the last two yards were draped over one shoulder. This afforded women enough modesty and was very practical for breastfeeding. But the idea that a woman's breast would be so readily available was a disgraceful thought to the foreigners. Women were taught how to sew (a nonexistent art in India before this time) in order that blouses could be made to cover and hide their breasts. If you venture into the remote villages even today, you will see women who escaped this edict.

> India lives in her villages.
> —*Mahatma Gandhi*

We often are very unsophisticated in thinking that what is acceptable behavior in one country or district is acceptable throughout the world. This is especially apparent in what we consider moral and appropriate sexual behavior. If it is not your belief, it may be difficult to reconcile yourself with the fact that in some parts of the world it is permissible to take on many husbands or wives. In some places you can take on one or more of each!

In the opening scene of John Patrick's *The Teahouse of the August Moon,* a very distinguished Japanese gentleman appears alone onstage. He bows and begins to address the audience of Americans. "In Okinawa . . . wash self in public bath with nude lady

quite proper. Picture of nude lady in private home . . . quite im-
proper. In America . . . statue of nude lady in park win prize. But
nude lady in flesh in park win penalty. Conclusion? Pornography
question of geography."

*Devoted to living a balanced and moderate life*
(**Brahmacharya**), *the scope of one's life force becomes*
*boundless.*

For millennia, yogis who knew the importance of balance, moderation, and redirecting sexual energy developed specific practices
for this purpose. They understood that we, like all of nature, ebb
and flow through cycles, sometimes needing to use our sexual energy and other times to preserve it. With the surge of puritanical
Western thinking, the dignity of moderation and balance became
distorted. This repression caused a rise in celibacy, driving many of
the sacred teachings underground. The path of celibacy was then
elevated as the zenith of spirituality and the quickest way to reach
the Divine.

One of the most detrimental consequences of this misinterpretation was the separation of spirit from nature. Women (representing nature) were rejected from spiritual communion. Up to this
time, the woman had been seen as the Shakti (manifesting energy)
without whom the man could not function!

## EXPLORING THE FOUR *ASHRAMAS,* OR STAGES, OF LIFE

According to the ancient ways, there were four stages of life that
one passed through, learning a variety of lessons and experiences in
each. They offered an expanding way of service to one's self, one's
family, the spiritual community (*satsang*), and the entire world.

Living in balance, each individual had a life span of one hundred years or more. It was considered to be the effect of using the life force wisely. Divided into four, each stage affords us the attributes and temperament befitting our development. While the exact span of years in each of the stages may vary, notice how they portray the yearning to change focus as we progress through life. Even practicing them inwardly propels us toward spiritual freedom.

*Brahmacharya:* A time celebrated for creativity, play, and study. This all-important time is spent gaining knowledge about your relationship to yourself, the world, and the Divine. It is a time to explore and set patterns as to where and how you want to direct your energy. Because it is not yet the time for intimate relationships, as sexual energy begins to mature, the vital energy is available for study and learning and introspection.

*Grihastha:* The time has come to explore the world and all her abundant gifts. Settling on a profession or trade, you now embrace a long-term loving relationship. The refined vital sexual energy that has been cherished is available in its wholesome form to lovingly pleasure another, and to create and nurture children.

*Vanaprasta:* Less time is spent on your profession; the children are grown and have children of their own. You and your partner still enjoy physical intimacy and find the earlier intensity has evolved into deep tenderness and devotion. As more leisure time is available, you long to spend it in spiritual practice and study.

*Sannyasa:* Letting go of worldly duties and desires, you are drawn more toward the spiritual than the physical world. Drawing inward, most of your treasured time is dedicated to service, study, and devotion of the Divine.

As we can see, the four *Ashramas* of life seemed to follow a very natural and productive pattern. Each person transitioned through the various stages in the order presented. Spirituality was never intended to be a separate addition to life; it *was* life. As one reached the *Sannyasa* phase of withdrawing from the world, it was as natural as a snake shedding its skin. Occasionally, a few men (and only men at the time) were called to renounce personal life at an earlier age. They would then choose to remain unmarried, thus allowing them to be free to serve all without prejudice or favor.

For centuries the origin of women's power has been a mystery to men, and they have done much to try to capture it though repression, possession, and various tedious sexual practices. As we respect and esteem the vital energy, we are humbled to realize it holds the power to create another human being.

If abstinence were the sure way to the Divine, many people throughout the world would be realized beings. Like so many practices, it is more in the essence than in the act. Engage in the pleasures of making love as *Karma Yoga*. Your only desire is to pleasure the other person, and their only desire is to pleasure you. Each is fulfilled and satisfied, and when we are satisfied, we are moderate and balanced.

**Devoted to living a balanced and moderate life (Brahmacharya), *the scope of one's life force becomes boundless.***

### EXPERIENCING MODERATION (*BRAHMACHARYA*) IN YOUR LIFE

*Are there certain areas in your life where you could be more moderate? It could be food, work, TV, and so on. Choose one at a time and begin to moderate its use. For this example we will use food.*

*If you are accustomed to eating three large meals a day and many snacks, begin to eat less at mealtimes and half as much when you snack. Instead of two handfuls of nuts, take one.*

*The tendency would be to eat only one meal and eliminate all snacks. That would swing the pendulum from one extreme to the other. Remember, the idea is to practice moderation. We already know how to be excessive!*

*Notice how much energy you feel after a few days.*

*Then you can progress to moderating TV watching or overworking.*

*Slowly begin to move though all the areas in your life until moderation is the norm.*

**II.39** *Acknowledging abundance* (Aparigraha), *we recognize the blessings in everything and gain insights into the purpose for our worldly existence.*

*Aparigraha* gives us the secret to earthly life. Take a moment to feel gratitude for the great blessings that surround you: the home you live in, the service you do in the world, the availability and quantity of food you have to eat. The riches also include your friends, your health, and the opportunity to dedicate time to know your own heart. Even when you acknowledge the bounty, is there still a lingering apprehension that part or all of it may be taken away? That the well might run dry? Just thinking that a resource is limited initiates fear, thereby lessening the joy in the present moment.

As a society, we enjoy luxuries that were not even awarded to the royalty of the past. They were not blessed with the simple comforts we now consider everyday requirements. Central heat and air-conditioning, indoor plumbing, or simply a knob to turn in order to cook our meals are often taken for granted. The next time you are called to nature in the middle of the night, be thankful it is as near as the next heated room.

As a nation, our façade of abundance is possible because of what we imaginatively call credit, which in reality is debt. Debt is what we *really* accumulate when we amass all the so-called necessities we could not possibly live without. This masquerade is facilitated by our engorged belief in propriety and greed. Creating a complex misunderstanding of the flow of abundance, we tend to overlook the premise that when money is owed, obligation is accrued. Most important, we have distracted ourselves from the true happiness within by impeding access into the spiritual vistas with material wants and needs. If we are able to live within the material energy allotted us and generously use the word "enough," abundance cascades in our direction. We become free.

## LET GO AND BE FREE

We all know and recite the phrase "Money cannot buy happiness," yet we often trade our peace and health for the material security necessary to sustain our escalating lifestyle. Spiritual wealth is the only wealth that sustains us, and when we venture deep within, we are all millionaires!

Life's ebb and flow brings things into our life and then out again. Even the slightest hesitation of holding impedes the flow. Our belief system has the ability to hinder or expand this flow of abundance. If you believe that material and spiritual blessings are infinite, a cornucopia awaits you. If, instead, you accept the bounty as limited, your hopes and dreams will shrink to those proportions.

Our habit of waste runs contrary to *Aparigraha*. If we really believed that this was our *last* meal, would we not savor the food we have on our plate? In our fear of not getting enough, we often take too much on our plates, only to throw away the leftovers. As a nation, we are great consumers and also great wasters. We may buy a dress for one occasion and never wear it again but keep it *just in case*. Or every few years we might buy a new car that is bigger than the last, with an engine that consumes greater quantities of fossil fuels. How much does this affect us?

Whoever shuts their ears to the cry of the poor will also cry out and not be answered.

—*Old Testament*

Some allow material possessions to easily come and go; it is their thoughts and ideas that are etched in stone. When you form an opinion of someone or something, how effortlessly can you allow that opinion to change? One of the most difficult things is for us to change our thoughts and ways. Even more difficult is for us to accept the change in others.

What is it that you lost that you are grieving for? What is it that you brought into this world that you have lost? Whatever you gained, you gained from this world. Whatever you lost, you lost to this world. What belongs to you today, belonged to someone else yesterday and will belong to someone else tomorrow.

—Bhagavad Gita

*Acknowledging abundance* (Aparigraha), *we recognize the blessings in everything and gain insights into the purpose for our worldly existence.*

## EXPERIENCING ABUNDANCE (*APARIGRAHA*) BY LETTING THINGS GO

*Clean out a drawer or a closet and give the contents to a worthy person or charity. An empty place allows for new things to abundantly fill your life.*

*Move this same idea to your datebook. Leave some time each week for the unexpected to happen. Invite surprise blessings to visit you.*

## EXPERIENCING GRATITUDE FOR YOUR ABUNDANCE (*APARIGRAHA*)

*Plan some time, perhaps at the holidays, to feed the homeless or to read to the sick or the elderly.*

*Notice and record any mental or emotional resistance.*

*Review the way you live your life and try to imagine for what purpose you are here on this earth.*

*Note how you feel after the experience.*

*Do you feel an expansiveness and an experience of gratitude that accompanies it? Perhaps so much so that you may want to make this kind of Seva (selfless service) a regular event in your life.*

# NIYAMA:
## Evolution Toward Harmony

FIVE INNER FACETS of *Asthaanga Yoga* are presented here as *Niyama*, allowing us to continue our journey inward toward wholeness and discovering our divinity.

*Through simplicity and continual refinement (Saucha), the body, thoughts, and emotions become clear reflections of the Self within.*

*Saucha reveals our joyful nature, and the yearning for knowing the Self blossoms.*

*When at peace and content with oneself and others (Santosha), supreme joy is celebrated.*

*Living life with zeal and sincerity, the purifying flame is ignited (Tapas), revealing the inner light.*

*Sacred study of the Divine through scripture, nature, and introspection (Swadhaya) guides us to the Supreme Self.*

*Through wholehearted dedication (Iswara Pranidhana), we become intoxicated with the Divine.*

II.40 *Through simplicity and continual refinement (Saucha), the body, thoughts, and emotions become clear reflections of the Self within.*

II.41 Saucha *reveals our joyful nature, and the yearning for knowing the Self blossoms.*

Through the practice of *Saucha* our flawless essence becomes the basis for the choices and directions we invite into our life.

Pure silver is a lucid and shiny metal. Unrefined, it appears ordinary, its luminescence hidden. The process requires the silversmith to boil the unrefined silver over the hottest flame. It is essential for her to fully attend to the molten silver during this tedious process. If the silver remains in the fire for a moment longer than necessary, it could be destroyed. The correct amount of time yields awesome beauty. How does the silversmith know when the silver is fully refined? When she can clearly see her image in it. *Saucha* recalls the simple and pure energy of youth that fostered healthy development on all levels of our being. The same longing for simplicity, though sometimes hindered, continues throughout our lifetime.

## PURIFICATION BY NATURE

Many cultures have ritualistic bathing practices to encourage the continuation of this lifelong refinement. Early-morning immersions in a holy river, often performed while repeating prayers, purify not only the body but the mind and emotions as well, so the light in the heart can be experienced. Baptism purifies the body so the blessed spirit within can shine. On a less esoteric level, the enrichment gained by soaking in a natural hot spring, sauna, or steam bath continues to delight many as it has throughout the ages.

Women's bodies naturally cycle through their own unique phases—ovulation, menstruation, conception, pregnancy, child-birth, menopause. These dramatic sequences symbolize the highly sophisticated ways our bodies stay vital and healthy. Unable to understand the purpose for these cleansing cycles, male authority figures distorted them, marking women unclean and tainted during certain times of the month. Firm rules were established to keep us from "contaminating" men or sacred objects. Rituals were devised to purify and sanitize us before we could be accepted into the larger society again.

Yet was that not the job our bodies had just completed? The act of menstruating itself is purification! Driven by natural forces, we are *different* from men, not tarnished or unclean. All this ostracism could have been avoided with the alluring knowledge that the only true purity is *in each heart*. We were framed by a misconception so great that even today, women are thought to be unclean during those "special" times!

Respect woman as my equal in creation as bearing the image of God.

—*Unknown*

*Through simplicity and continual refinement* (Saucha), *the body, thoughts, and emotions become clear reflections of the Self within.*

Saucha *reveals our joyful nature, and the yearning for knowing the Self blossoms.*

## EVERYTHING IS HOLY TO THOSE WITH AN OPEN HEART

Nurses are the angels of mercy in the medical profession. They serve with compassion and take their rewards from knowing they bring comfort and healing to us. Often they have the unpleasant duty of cleaning up bodily discharges. It is their purity of heart that allows them to serve us at our greatest and most humbling time of need without judgment or aversion.

The illustrious Florence Nightingale formalized the nursing profession. Abandoning her privilege and status, she chose to dedicate her life to the sick and infirm. The essence of compassion, "the lady with the lamp" selflessly spent long hours bringing comfort to many. She revolutionized hospital care with simple yet essential improvements. Basic procedures we now take for granted, such as keeping the body washed and dressings clean and placing a bell at the bedside allowed patients dignity in the face of distress.

Mother Teresa of Calcutta many years later exemplified Florence Nightingale's basic principles. Encountering the destitute and the sick lying on the streets, she cradled them in her arms, impervious to the unsanitary condition of their bodies, offering them a moment of love and dignity before they died.

When difficulties would arise during our healing retreats for those with cancer, Mother Teresa's words returned to inspire me: "The miracle is not that we do this work. The miracle is that we *love* to do this work."

## NOT-SO-OBVIOUS SIMPLICITY

Cultivating simplicity of mind and emotions can be a refreshing change from the complicated world we live in.

When American scientists were making plans to send the first human into weightless space, they encountered many challenges that gravity-bound Earth did not have. Something as routine as keeping a log facilitated the invention of a special writing instrument. In normal usage, ink flows downward from the pen to the paper. This is all done with the persistent force of gravity. Without this force, the ink floats any which way, making writing impossible. Finally, millions of dollars in research and development yielded a pen that could do the job of writing in zero gravity. The ship's logs could now be filled in. The Russians, however, took the simpler route and saved an enormous amount of money. They used a pencil!

It is truly a "gift to be simple." The blessings come when we can embrace simplicity, making our lives easier and more joyous. *Saucha* is the purity deep within our own heart that resonates as our guide to knowing.

> Blessed are the pure in heart, for they shall see God.
>
> —*New Testament*

Another aspect of *Saucha* is the ability to be emotionally light. We tend to take situations and ourselves much too seriously. Observing the humor in life promotes emotional purity.

> Creator—A comedian whose audience is afraid to laugh.
>
> —*H. L. Mencken*

*Through simplicity and continual refinement* (Saucha), *the body, thoughts, and emotions become clear reflections of the Self within.*

Saucha *reveals our joyful nature, and the yearning for knowing the Self blossoms.*

## EXPERIENCING THE POWER OF PURITY AND SIMPLICITY (*SAUCHA*)

*Observe how your body changes with the different foods you eat. If the weather is hot and you eat spicy or warming foods, notice if your body perspires more than it does when you consume cool foods or drinks.*

*When watching a scary movie or reading a disturbing book, notice how your thoughts and emotions mimic that mood. It could be an immediate response, or it could be a delayed one in a totally different situation.*

*Are there certain clothes or surroundings that allow you to feel a sense of refinement in your being?*

*When you walk on a pristine beach, or in a forest, does the simplicity of nature afford the mind and emotions a joyful feeling? Does it seem like all the worries you brought with you surrender to the peaceful surroundings?*

*Write down which foods, clothes, and places allow you to feel that sense of purity, simplicity, and refinement. How do they assist you in feeling that way? The next time you are deciding what to eat, what to wear, or where to visit, recall what feeling you want to evoke and then follow its lead in choosing.*

*When you are involved in a stressful situation, try to look at it another way, finding a bit of humor that can lighten the mood. Laughter allows the heart to blossom.*

## II.42 *When at peace and content with oneself and others* (Santosha), *supreme joy is celebrated.*

*Santosha* is an agreement of faith that we make with our Divine Self. This faith fastens us to the peace that abides in our hearts, no matter what the Fates bring. By this affirmation we firmly identify with our inner essence rather than with external objects. Our identification then travels with gratitude, appreciating how much we have rather than how much we want. With this attitude, all things that come and go do not have the opportunity to override our joy. Instead, they metamorphose into stillness and peace.

## KEEPING YOUR HEART LIGHT AS A FEATHER

In ancient Egypt, after the death of a pharaoh, the heart was removed from the body to be measured against the weight of a feather. If the heart was found to be heavier than the feather's weight, the monarch was considered not ready for admission to heaven. The scale, although normally the measure of physical weight, was thought to reveal the degree of emotional heaviness held in the heart. The *lighthearted* were presumably permitted entry through a special ritual, as their physical heart was given a place of honor in the burial plot.

> Content with an ordinary life, you can show all people the way back to their own true nature.
>
> —*Lao-tzu*

*When at peace and content with oneself and others* (Santosha), *supreme joy is celebrated.*

## JOY IS ACCEPTING WHAT IS

Some of us open naturally to joy, while others need to cultivate it more carefully. For most of us, the subtler aspects of *Santosha* elude us from time to time. Everlasting joy cleaves to us through our cultivating the understanding that we hold the power to our happiness. Even if temporarily lost, our joy will soon return, as it is the lifelong reward for attaining wisdom.

In South India there is a heartfelt way of expressing one's appreciation. Instead of saying "thank you," they say "*Santosha* [I am content]."

**When at peace and content with oneself and others (Santosha), supreme joy is celebrated.**

### EXPERIENCING YOUR JOYFUL NATURE

*Venture to a comfortable place, either physically or in your imagination, where the surroundings evoke a feeling of peace and joy.*

*Spend a few minutes experiencing comfort with the ambiance and notice if you spontaneously begin to smile.*

*Once the smile forms, let it engrave on your face, close your eyes, and journey inward.*

*Notice how the outer smile is greeted by the inner smile of contentment in your heart.*

*The smile is the outward expression of the joy.*

*When you leave the physical place that invoked this feeling, the outward smile remains as the constant reminder of your inner*

*contentment. Sharing it with each person you meet is like shar-*
*ing a place in your heart.*

*If at any time the contentment seems to be hiding, coax it out*
*with a sweet upturning of your lips and cheeks and a sparkle in*
*your eyes.*

## II.43 *Living life with zeal and sincerity, the purifying flame is ignited (*Tapas*), revealing the inner light.*

Once again we visit *Tapas, Swadhaya,* and *Iswara Pranidhana,* which complemented one another as *Kriya Yoga,* sutra II.1. This time they are woven into *Asthaanga Yoga* as the final three *Niyamas.* Their importance is reinforced by their repetition in the sutras.

### *TAPAS* OF BODY, MIND, AND SPEECH

The Bhagavad Gita speaks to us of *Tapas,* kindling the purify-ing flame through refining the actions of our bodies, minds, and speech.

*Tapas of body* is defined as service, physical purity, living in vir-tue, moderation, and reverence for all.

Charging all your actions with zeal and sincerity—whether serv-ing family, the greater community, or yourself—transforms them into spiritual practice. This concept applies to the formal practices as well. When practicing *Asana* (posture), *Pranayama* (guidance of universal energy), or any of the other practices, the main benefit comes from embracing the deep spiritual intention.

*Tapas of mind* is distinguished as tranquil, gentle, kind, and quiet and involves willpower and purity of thought.

How we think and feel is a predictor of our physical health and vitality. Our relationships with the world around us are molded by the way we *imagine* them to be. By keeping our mind tranquil, gentle, and pure, we create a life worthy of spiritual reflection.

*Tapas of speech* is experienced as truthful, pleasant, serene, and beneficial and involves prayer and *japa* (repetition of a mantra).

Speech is a direct outward expression of the mind and emotions. If we are agitated or upset, our language mimics that point of view. Consciously choosing words that are pleasant and serene, we are able to *influence* the mind and emotions into calmness. Prayer and mantra are ways of extending the vistas of our speech to reach the place where all understanding resides.

This clear, threefold description of *Tapas* from the Bhagavad Gita allows us the liberty to experience varied ways of transforming energy. When the practices are not separate from but incorporated into our lives, the unfolding of our hearts continues. The Bhagavad Gita assures us that it is not necessary to engage in rigorous practices; these steady and subtle ways slowly ignite the spark of divinity within our heart.

While there are varied forms of sacrifice one can make with zeal and sincerity, simple acts of devotion, whether private or public, have powerful and lasting effects.

**Living life with zeal and sincerity, the purifying flame is ignited (Tapas), *revealing the inner light*.**

## AN EXQUISITE TEST OF FAITH

The brilliant poet Maya Angelou talked with passion and tenderness of one of her fiercest tests and how she ascended to a high level of understanding through sacred prayer. (This story beautifully illustrates the perfect blending of *Tapas, Swadhaya,* and *Iswara Pranidhana.*)

An alarming phone call revealed that her precious son was hospitalized and not expected to live. "Could you come quickly?" the frightened voice asked. She could hardly have arrived more quickly if she had the power to materialize at will.

The doctors were confident that her son would live only a short time longer. Hearing that proclamation, she enjoined everyone concerned to convey *only positive thoughts* when entering her son's hospital room. Summoning all her faith and strength, she began a prayer vigil that, she vowed, would continue until her son had made *a total recovery.* She would consider no other outcome. Her heart and soul entwined in chorus, "God, I am thanking you in advance for the full recovery of my son." Her prayer was clear and simple, leaving not even a hair's breadth for doubt or confusion.

Moving from the seed in her heart, the prayer flooded her mind, giving it voice. "God, I am thanking you in advance for the full recovery of my son." Over and over she prayed, in a heart-wrenching refrain that summoned compassion from all the angels, "God, I am thanking you in advance for the full recovery of my son." All through the night, aware of nothing else, her powerful voice echoed through the room and up to the heavens. Drawn by her sincerity and passion, many joined her in chorus, "God, I am thanking you in advance for the full recovery of my son." As others tired and left, she continued until she *knew* that the prayers were being heard. "God, I am thanking you in advance for the full recovery of my son." At times her voice started to waver, but never her heart.

Not until her son returned from the coma to a semiwaking state did she even begin to slow down her vigil. After the full recovery of her son, she was asked if she ever doubted that her prayers would be answered. "If doubt even started to peek its head up, I'd bellow even louder. The Good Lord might have been busy and I wanted to make sure He could hear me. And I kept the prayer going for weeks after. I was not satisfied until my son *fully recovered.*"

I have an inward treasure born within me, which can keep me alive if all the extraneous delights should be withheld; or offered only at a price I cannot afford.

—*Charlotte Brontë*

*Living life with zeal and sincerity, the purifying flame is ignited* (**Tapas**), *revealing the inner light.*

## EXPERIENCING LIVING YOUR LIFE WITH ZEAL AND SINCERITY

*Choose the* Tapas of speech *from the* Bhagavad Gita *as the focus of your practice. Notice how your voice resonates and observe the choice of words you use.*

*For a revealing look at this, take a small recording device and place it under a table or out of sight the next time you visit with a friend. Turn it on at the outset of your conversation. Soon you will forget it is there.*

*After your friend leaves, listen to your words and expressions. Was your speech tranquil and gentle? Did it bring benefit to yourself and your friend?*

*How was the tone of your voice? Did you feel soothed or agitated listening to yourself?*

*Was it enlightening to listen to yourself speaking (if perhaps a bit intimidating)?*

> *Incorporate the positive changes you would like to introduce into your speech for a week and repeat the process.*
>
> *Continue refining and, after some time, you will find the outer speech reflects not only the mind and emotions but your heart as well.*

## II.44 *Sacred study of the Divine through scripture, nature, and introspection* (Swadhaya) *guides us to the Supreme Self.*

*Swadhaya* guides us to know ourselves through outward observation *and* inner reflection. Often we experience an incomprehensible phenomenon, either in nature or within our minds and hearts. If we are unable to understand it intuitively, we seek external sources. If, for example, we seek understanding of the movements of the tides or the cycles of the moon, we may consult an astronomer and conduct a thorough investigation of how gravity works.

However, if seeking a spiritual understanding, finding an outside source becomes a more delicate matter. It may take days, weeks, or longer to find a holy book or a teacher to assuage doubts or endorse experiences. Why is it we are able to learn so much from some people and have great difficulty learning from others? Is it their ability to quote great teachings or the grace they exude that transports us to the depth of understanding, or perhaps something deeper still?

One such great teacher, a revered and noble rabbi, had breathed his last breath, leaving the congregation in soulful mourning. An outsider became curious about this esteemed rabbi who drew such veneration on his death. He began interviewing a few of the close disciples who were blessed to have studied with the rabbi. The refrains were varied and vague. "I cannot exactly say how he inspired me; we learned the teachings through his discourses, but more was transmitted by the way he lived his life." "He was a very humble man." One disciple sitting off by himself, his eyes brimming with tears, whispered softly, "I used to love to watch the way, with great reverence, he took off his shoes."

> Study brings us wisdom, wisdom brings us life.
>
> —*Rabbi Hillel*

We tend to revere book learning in these times, overstuffing our minds with all kinds of information. If you read one Sunday issue of *The New York Times* cover to cover, you have exposed yourself to more information than the average person one hundred years ago read during her or his entire lifetime!

## FACT TODAY, FICTION TOMORROW

We often forget that observing natural occurrences has made many important discoveries. Alexander Fleming's curiosity led him to study a simple mold, offensive to most of us, making the intuitive leap that these organisms could miraculously cure infection. Commonly known as penicillin, the minute spores became the panacea that saved millions of lives.

Many theories may be correct and accurate today, but tomorrow, with new discoveries and advancements, those "truths" of yesterday may be discounted. What happens to our belief in the first theory? Is it shaken? The mind wants to switch to the new hypothesis, but how quickly are we able to change?

Several hundred years ago, a few noble scientists, including Giordano Bruno, proclaimed that the Earth was not the center of the planetary system, let alone the universe! The repercussions were uproarious, and the theory was considered blasphemous. It was a well-known *fact* at that time that the sun, as well as all the other planets, orbited around the Earth! The outraged church declared the discovery to be heresy. Bruno, a prominent astronomer, a seer, and a speaker of truth, was burned at the stake.

Later, Galileo corroborated Bruno's theory and was sentenced to house arrest for the remainder of his life. Today the idea that the Earth revolves around the sun is a straightforward observation (we even call it the solar system), a statement of fact, but at that time the opposite was considered *truth*.

We all agree that the Earth revolves around the sun; yet we continue to use archaic language. What words do you use to describe what you observe at dawn and dusk? Do you say the sun *rises* in the morning and *sets* in the evening? Most people do. Yet we just clearly established that the sun does not revolve around us, so how could it rise and set? Even with correct knowledge, we are slow to change our consciousness and our metaphors.

Always be willing for your concept of reality to change as your consciousness brightens.

*Sacred study of the Divine through scripture, nature, and introspection* (Swadhaya) *guides us to the Supreme Self.*

### EXPERIENCING THE ROTATION OF THE EARTH AND CHANGING YOUR CONCEPT OF SUNRISE AND SUNSET

*Sit or stand comfortably with a clear view of the sky at predawn or predusk.*

*Observe the sun and notice how your mind travels to the customary yet erroneous relationship between the sun and the*

Earth. While your deep thoughts hold the truth, the habitual mind holds the notion that the sun rises and sets while you, planted on the Earth, remain stationary.

Become very quiet and begin to imagine that you and the Earth are actually moving either toward the sun (dawn) or away from the sun (dusk). Notice how your mind will try to resist this phenomenon.

After a time, you may be able to feel the steady, slow motion. You may even get a bit dizzy.

It may take a while, but as you repeat this observation, the flow will seem more natural. Then the challenge will be to come up with other terminology for the Earth's movements, letting go of the terms "sunrise" and "sunset."

Use the same principles with other concepts that you may believe to be so.

Look to a learned source for affirmation and challenge yourself to change!

## 11.45 *Through wholehearted dedication* (Iswara Pranidhana), *we become intoxicated with the Divine.*

For the third time in the sacred sutras, *Iswara Pranidhana* is encouraging us to live with wholehearted devotion to the Divine and divine creation. As *Ahimsa* is the pinnacle from which all of the *Yamas* flow, *Iswara Pranidhana* is the zenith of the *Niyamas*.

Devotion is the key to unlocking our hearts. When living with an open heart, we see clearly as the pathways of our lives unfold. Faith allows us to trust in the present moment as we observe our part in the divine plan.

Love and devotion can be expressed as a simple blessing we bestow on ourselves or others, such as saying "Bless you" when someone sneezes. Often prayers invoke a higher source for something as mundane as losing our keys: "Please, Divine Mother, help me find my keys."

## MANY WAYS TO PRAY TO THE ONE

Prayers come in as many forms as there are hearts to recite them. Here are a few of the more traditional ways prayer is summoned:

*Petition:* appeals to the Divine to fulfill our needs or wishes (*"Divine Mother, please help me get this job"*).

*Intercession:* pleas made on behalf of another (*"Divine Mother, please let my daughter get into college"*).

*Thanksgiving:* expressions of deep gratitude (*"Thank you, Divine Mother, for allowing our home to be saved from the fire"*).

*Praise:* glorification of the Divine and creation (*"Blessed be you who made this beautiful day"*).

*Blessings:* invoking the Divine Grace to bless, protect, and guide us and others (*"Divine Mother, please bless and protect our family through this time of great trial"*).

*Affirmation:* heartfelt expression of the uncertainty of our faith in the divine plan of the universe (*"Divine Mother, I do not understand why this great sorrow is upon us; please give me the faith and strength to withstand it and keep my trust in you strong"*).

> More things are wrought by prayer than this world dreams of.
> —*Alfred, Lord Tennyson*

*Through wholehearted dedication* (Iswara Pranidhana), *we become intoxicated with the Divine.*

Prayers can be directed to the Divine within or to an outward presence. Much of the time we go back and forth according to the moment and mood. Most of us summon the greatest power of prayer in difficult times. When all other avenues have been exhausted and the enormity of the situation becomes too great to bear alone, we then pray to someone else out there as a separate person or manifestation to help us cope. We are really just summoning all the positive energy and celestial beings that are standing by to make our lives easier in all ways. Extending and reaching our arms toward the sky, we surrender in prayer.

It is preferable to cultivate faith and devotion *before* we are in desperate need. Wholehearted devotion connects us through faith to our source. Learning to trust the power within, we courageously let go and live each moment to the fullest. That, after all, is how life is doled out to us, one moment at a time. We then become intoxicated with the Divine.

> Come to the edge.
> We might fall.
> Come to the edge.
> It's too high!
> COME TO THE EDGE!
> And they came
> and he pushed
> and they flew . . .
>
> —*Christopher Logue*

*Through wholehearted dedication* (Iswara Pranidhana), *we become intoxicated with the Divine.*

## EXPERIENCING THE POWER OF WHOLEHEARTED DEDICATED (*ISWARA PRANIDHANA*) PRAYER

*Notice the times when you feel the desire to pray. Is it at times of joy or times of unhappiness? If your prayers are always petitions, try reforming them to express gratitude.*

*If you use praise, feeling you will receive something in return, affirm that blessings are abundant.*

*Begin to formulate an affirmation or prayer in your own words that allows you to expand into the next level of joy.*

*Repeat this prayer or affirmation at first at "formal" times in the morning and evening. Then begin to repeat it as many times during the day as possible, encouraging the repetition in both your mind and heart.*

*To help you to remember this gem during the day, place a colored dot on your watch, or a note on the computer, the telephone, the car ignition, or anyplace you frequent. Let it be a constant reminder, as you glance at it, to remember and repeat the affirmation or prayer.*

*In a week's time, change the wording to reflect yet another layer of your divinity. Continue to grow and blossom as the joy comes forth.*

# HATHA YOGA:
## Harmonizing Body, Breath, and Senses

W E NOW EXPERIENCE how the outward harmony of body, breath, and senses reveals our inner nature.

*The natural comfort and joy of our being is expressed when the body becomes steady (Asana).*

*As the body yields all efforts and holdings, the infinite within is revealed.*

*Thereafter we are freed from the fluctuations of the gunas.*

*The universal life force (prana) is enhanced and guided through the harmonious rhythm of the breath (Pranayama).*

*The movement of the life force is influenced by inhalation, exhalation, and sustained breath.*

*A balanced, rhythmic pattern steadies the mind and emotions, causing the breath to become motionless.*

*As a result, the veils over the inner light are lifted.*

*The vista of higher consciousness is revealed.*

*Encouraging the senses to draw inward is*
Pratyahara.

*Glimpsing the inner light, the senses contentedly dwell within.*

II.46 *The natural comfort and joy of our being is expressed when the body becomes steady* (Asana).

II.47 *As the body yields all efforts and holdings, the infinite within is revealed.*

II.48 *Thereafter we are freed from the fluctuations of the* gunas.

The *Yama* and *Niyama* enable us to model the attitudes of Golden Age consciousness. We now venture to the next three facets of *Asthaanga Yoga,* known as *Hatha Yoga.* Their positioning after *Yama* and *Niyama* suggests that embracing a high level of behavior before beginning asana practice protects us from misusing or wasting the very powerful energy that is released. When we are firmly grounded in these principles, any unseemly thoughts or emotions are neither exacerbated nor strengthened.

## HA-THA —A BALANCE OF ENERGIES

The complete system of *Hatha Yoga* increases vital energy by aligning our physical and subtle bodies through physical poses (*Asana*), guiding and enhancing the life force through breathing practices (*Pranayama*), and encouraging the senses inward through deep relaxation (*Pratyahara*). All three aspects were designed to be practiced in concert, thereby harmonizing body, breath, and senses.

When popularized in the West, the physical postures were isolated, excluding the other two aspects of *Hatha Yoga* almost completely. This oversight can encourage imbalances and injuries to the body, as well as to the mental and emotional well-being. Today most people commonly refer to the isolated practice of *Asana* as the total system, simply calling it Yoga.

*Hatha* represents the integrated energy that then polarizes within each of us as light and dark, sun and moon, masculine and feminine. *Ha* represents the sun, heating, and "masculine" qualities of reason and intellectual thinking, while *tha* characterizes the moon, cooling, and "feminine" qualities of emotional and intuitive feelings. Each one of us has both the male *ha* and the female *tha* within us in varied proportions. The finer the balance, the more harmonious we feel.

When describing *Asana,* sutra II.46 uses two Sanskrit words: *sthira* and *sukha.*

*Sthira* denotes an effortlessness while coming into the pose or posture, holding it, or coming out of it.

*Sukha* reflects the natural state of comfort and joy. As the body finds its ease, the mind and emotions align with it, reflecting the light of the Divine. It allows us the feeling of being comfortable in our own skin. The inner and outer worlds interconnect.

The placement of the sutras in *Hatha Yoga* suggests they are a preparation for sitting meditation. Aching bodies distracted the ancient yogis in their quest to sit still. Unable to dedicate their focus inward, they realized that settling the mind was unlikely if even the slightest distraction remained in the body.

By practicing a few simple poses *before* sitting, you encourage a sense of comfort and ease in the body, the mind calms, and the spirit is more readily accessed. After all, a certain amount of discipline and physical strength is needed to keep the body in a steady seated position without movement for a half hour or longer. Through *Asana* practice, distractions of the body become infrequent visitors. The result is that we feel better, look better, and can project that feeling into our daily life.

The practice of *Asana* encourages the body, mind, and breath to function together. The mind first decides on the movement and then directs the energy. The physical body, given the blueprint, follows. Much of our pain, stiffness, and disease is caused by the low quantity or impeded flow of energy in the body and mind.

Rhythmic breathing coordinated with this movement releases blockages and allows energy to flow. Holding the breath gives our nervous system a distress signal that is then sent to the organs, glands, and muscular system. When it is flowing normally and rhythmically, the breath distributes energy through pathways, which encourages relaxation and the ability to stretch further.

Along with bringing ease to the body, the practice of *Asana* was intended by the *sadhus* (spiritual seekers) to prepare their bodies for the intense physical rigor that was a fact of their lives. It was a very different time and culture from ours. When the practice of *Asana* traversed the world, the need to adapt the poses for Western bodies became apparent. For example, from childhood to old age in most Asian countries, people commonly sit in a simple cross-legged pose. For them it is quite comfortable. If we at age thirty, forty, or fifty try to adapt that same simple pose, our knees may complain for days or longer afterward. When the adaptations are not heeded, we find the asanas difficult to do well and often, and the benefits will be overshadowed by frustration or injury.

## THE FEMININE UNIQUENESS

It is also an important distinction to note that the asanas were designed for the needs of a male body. A woman's body and her emotional makeup have unique qualities that need special attention. Many of the poses need to be adapted to the female body. Yet our special needs are ignored if we follow traditional *Asana* instruction rather than our intuition. While gentle pressure and squeezing help to improve blood circulation and health, too-vigorous bending and stretching can harm the softer and less muscular female body.

I would always joke with my students when teaching the *mayurasana,* or peacock, pose. In this pose, the entire weight of the body is balanced on bent arms as the elbows push into the belly so the straightened legs can be raised into the air. In order to accomplish this pose, the balance point must be at the center of the body (the elbows being the fulcrum). But the female pelvis is bigger and heavier than a man's, making the center of gravity lower. So if, adhering to the traditional instructions, the elbows are pushed into the abdomen, most women would fall forward and flat on their faces when they raised their legs. By pushing the elbows into the pelvis rather than the abdomen, we are more easily able to balance. However, while the elbows against the pelvis enable us to do the pose, they can put too much pressure on the delicate organs housed there. Injury or imbalance can occur. Since the position mimics a peacock (male) with long tail feathers splayed, I suggest women do a version I call peahen pose, in which the legs are folded and tucked underneath the belly. In this way, the center of gravity shifts and the pose is accomplished.

The mental, emotional, and energetic aspects of *Asana* can be as great as if not greater than the physical aspect. When the mind imagines the benefits of a pose, the energy moves more easily to that part. Then we receive maximum benefits from the practice—a relaxed, healthy body and mind. All this stretching leads us to a supple body of health and strength that is able to be active as well as to sit perfectly still.

On an emotional level, a woman's sensitivity often shifts to more of a masculine *ha* if she continually takes on challenges and engages in competition. Instead of experiencing feelings of compassion when confronted with a situation, we may first exhibit anger. Because of the emphasis placed on our more masculine side, our feminine qualities are depleted instead of enhanced. Both aspects need to be honored.

Today there are hundreds of methods and schools for practicing

Yoga poses. Choose the type of *Asana* you want to practice, based not just on the physical benefits but also on how it will affect your emotional makeup. It is essential to understand what type of practice your particular temperament requires. Also, be aware of the effect that the practice is having on the subtle nervous system. If your nervous system is sensitive and you adopt a vigorous *Asana* practice, it may cause an imbalance. Allow *Asana* to be one part of your complete *Hatha Yoga* practice.

As the practice is established, it affords flexibility of body, mind, and emotions. With this comes balance and the yearning to be still and know yourself.

The body itself is to reveal the light that's blazing inside your Presence.

—*Rumi*

*The natural comfort and joy of our being is expressed when the body becomes steady* (Asana).

*As the body yields all efforts and holdings, the infinite within is revealed.*

*Thereafter we are freed from the fluctuations of the* gunas.

### EXPERIENCING HOW THOUGHT INFLUENCES THE FLEXIBILITY OF THE BODY

*Choose two asanas that you are familiar with, one that you can do with ease and love and one that is a little more challenging for your body.*

*Begin to practice the one you love and notice why you like it. Is it because you are proficient at it, or does it just feel good?*

*Notice how the mind and the feelings react after you have fin-
ished.*

*Invoke the same happy feeling that came to you during the asana
you love. Hold that feeling and transpose it on the other asana.
If the mind starts to move into "I cannot do this well; I really do
not like the way this one makes me feel," then bring the mind
back to the happy feeling.*

*Soon you may experience a release replaced by a feeling of com-
fort and ease of the body that just a few moments before had
seemed impossible.*

**II.49** *The universal life force* (prana) *is enhanced and
guided through the harmonious rhythm of the breath*
(Pranayama).

**II.50** *The movement of the life force is influenced by
inhalation, exhalation, and sustained breath.*

Inhabiting and surrounding each cell of our physical body is the
universal energy called *prana* (this energy is named *qi* in Japan and
*chi* in China). Everything in the natural world has a field of energy
surrounding and circulating through it. At different times the quality and quantity of *prana* may vary.

For example, a tree in winter would have less circulating *prana*
than a tree in springtime. There is more energy needed for a tree to
flower than to exist in the dormant stage. *Prana* is the intelligence

that responds to the varying needs. *Prana* is similar to electricity in that it supplies an invisible current to keep life flowing and functioning.

At birth, we are allotted a quantity of this precious vital energy that continuously circulates, maintaining our function in daily life. Our first life-affirming action on this planet is to inhale, taking in the precious atmosphere of the earth, as well as a dose of *prana*. This action enlivens our bodies, making them suitable to sustain life in our new world. We then continue to breathe about sixteen times a minute, hopefully for many years to come. At a certain time, very near the last beat of our hearts, we return the borrowed air we took in at the beginning with an exhalation and go on our way, out of our body and to our next destination. In this way a breathing body is considered to be alive, and a breathless body is considered to be dead. What is often overlooked is that we are the indweller of the body, not the body itself.

While a substantial portion of *prana* is allotted for daily use, a greater amount is put "in trust" until the time comes to further our quest to know the Divine Self. A vast capacity of *prana* is needed to raise the energy from the physical to the spiritual realms. This "trust fund" is safely stored at the base of the spine, most often known as the *Kundalini* (coiled snake). Through the wide range of yogic practices, we slowly access this energy as it guides us to deeper levels of consciousness.

Our senses augment the already-circulating *prana*: Through the beauty, we see; the sounds, we hear; the touch, we receive; the fragrance, we smell; the food, we eat. The sun, moon, stars, thoughts, emotions, actions, and words all have the capacity to enhance or diminish our *prana*.

## THE SUBTLE NERVOUS SYSTEM

It is estimated that there are between 75,000 and 150,000 subtle pathways, or *nadis,* within and surrounding the physical body. The purpose of these *nadis* is to circulate and distribute the much-needed energy to the physical, mental, and emotional bodies (*koshas*). The *nadis* function in a similar way to the blood vessels. Of the many thousand of *nadis,* three are most significant: *Ida, Pingala,* and *Shushumna.*

The *Pingala nadi* and *Ida nadi* polarize the neutral energy as they wind around the spinal cord. The *prana* circulates through the *Pingala nadi* (the *ha,* or sun, in *Hatha*), generating heat and the masculine attributes of rational thinking and intellectual reasoning. The *Pingala* governs the sympathetic nervous system and corresponds to the left side of the brain.

When *prana* circulates through the *Ida nadi* (the *tha,* or moon, in *Hatha*), it produces a coolness and accesses the feminine attributes of emotion, feelings, and intuition. *Ida* guides the parasympathetic nervous system and corresponds with the right side of the brain.

The *Shushumna nadi* comes into play only when the *Pingala* and *Ida* are in perfect harmony. It then has the sacred duty to carry the *prana* through to the higher centers of consciousness (chakras). It does not function as the day-to-day distributor of energy to the physical, mental, or emotional bodies.

*The universal life force* (prana) *is enhanced and guided through the harmonious rhythm of the breath* (Pranayama).

*The movement of the life force is influenced by inhalation, exhalation, and sustained breath.*

This refined circulation of *prana* is possible because of our sophisticated system of breathing, which facilitates this process much as the pumping heart does for the circulatory system. Through the steady rhythm of inhalation (*Puraka*) and exhalation (*Rechaka*), the air and *prana* circulate within and between the physical and subtle bodies. The inhalation draws the *prana* to the center of our being, and with the exhalation it journeys outward. All this happens within the breath's regular pattern of sixteen times a minute. A slight hesitation (*Kumbaka*) between the inhalation and the exhalation allows oxygen as well as the precious *prana* to be distributed.

## THE CHANGING PATTERNS

Having two nostrils supports the flow of energy through *Pingala* and *Ida*. Although most of us are probably unaware of it, the lining of each nostril engorges and shrinks periodically during the day. This shifts the flow of air from one nostril to the other in a biological rhythm. Every one and a half to three hours, the *Pingala* and the *Ida* alternate dominance, in hopes of restoring balance. Extreme heat or cold can also cause the nostrils to change or switch dominance. Allowing the air to pass through the right or left nostril produces a heating or cooling effect, respectively. Outside on a cold winter's day—even though you are not aware of it—your right nostril is fully open and desperately trying to heat the body. When the environment suddenly changes as you walk into an overheated room, your right nostril will occlude, and the left will go on duty. This alternating pattern becomes more obvious when you have a head cold that stuffs up your nose. Usually one of the nostrils opens just enough to let some air flow through. When both nostrils are completely clogged, we resort to using the only viable alternative, the mouth, to breathe.

All of our physical systems depend on the regular flow of air *and* of *prana*. If our habitual breathing patterns are upset or halted because of erratic movements in our body, the oxygen and energy requirements go up. If we suddenly run or quicken our pace, the breath accelerates, using up more *prana*. As we slow down, our breath follows.

If our bodies can change our breathing pattern, then the opposite is also true. A deep breath revitalizes us when we are tired. When we observe how these variations in breathing change our breathing according to our daily functions and moods, *Pranayama* becomes an essential practice in returning us to balance.

Mental states affect the breathing pattern and also change nostril dominance. When we feel anger or passion, which are heating emotions, chances are our right nostril will be open. Depression or a sense of quietness may cause the left nostril to take over. At night, as the nostril dominance shifts, we turn from one side to the other. Whichever side we are lying on, the opposite nostril is open. If you nap in the heat of day, the left nostril's vigilance allows you to rest deeply. If, suddenly, the phone rings, disturbing your sleep, the left nostril will engorge, causing the right nostril to release and allowing you to be present for the call. The body's consciousness is awake even when we are sleeping.

The mind and emotions host millions of thoughts and feelings that are perpetually hungry for energy in order to move about and function. These thoughts and feelings respond to the same rhythmic relationship the breath has with the body. With a long, slow exhalation, they have room to spread out. The measured, rhythmic pace allows them time to consider whether and how they will manifest. This is similar to the spacing of notes in music. The greater the spacing between the notes, the more relaxing effect the music produces. Awareness of the breath can boost the enjoyment and vitality of each moment of life.

When a balance between the *Pingala* and the *Ida* is sustained over a period of time through various *Pranayama* practices, the *prana* is then directed through the central *nadi, the Shushumna.* This centers the mind and emotions, moving beyond their grasp propelling us toward the highest consciousness (*Samadhi*).

*The universal life force* (prana) *is enhanced and guided through the harmonious rhythm of the breath* (Pranayama).

*The movement of the life force is influenced by inhalation, exhalation, and sustained breath.*

## MAGNETIZE YOURSELF TOWARD BALANCE AND HARMONY

Taking in a deep breath has the effect of "combing" our energy. When we visit the mirror after we wake up, we usually see that our hair is in disarray. We're unfazed, since we learned early on that a strategically placed comb or brush could coax the hairs to go more or less in the same direction. Satisfied, we look and feel a bit more in control (at least of our hair!). Breathing practices have the same effect on our energy field, our *pranic* body. With rhythmic breathing, we align and "comb" the energy; it becomes smoother, calmer, and more focused. This focused energy then acts like a magnet, attracting like polarities to us.

In a plain piece of metal, all the molecules are in chaos, facing every which way. A magnet is a similar piece of metal in which all the molecules are perfectly aligned—the north poles facing one way, and the south poles facing in the opposite direction. Because of this alignment, the magnet gains the power to attract and hold other objects. If you stroke the ordinary metal and the magnet together in one direction only, the magnet will align all the molecules in the plain metal with itself, causing a second magnet to emerge. The power to attract and hold has been transmitted from one to the other, while amazingly enough, the original magnet retains its full strength. If you now take the two magnets and stroke them so the repelling poles are facing each other, the strength of each will diminish. The power to attract and hold is gone. We can see the benefit of being with those that support us rather than neutralize our power (*satsang*).

*The universal life force* (prana) *is enhanced and guided through the harmonious rhythm of the breath* (Pranayama).

*The movement of the life force is influenced by inhalation, exhalation, and sustained breath.*

As we align our energies in this way, through regulating the breath, we maintain calm through the ordinary emotional roller-coaster rides we encounter each day. We find that when we are upset, everything around us reflects the same disturbance, as if it were somehow contagious. When tranquility prevails, it magnetizes everything with the same sense of calmness.

## BREATH, MIND, AND EMOTIONS IN HARMONY

Children allow us to see how our thoughts and emotions are linked with the breath. When they become frightened, their breath and speech patterns change. Often they will come running in breathlessly to tell us of some disturbing event that happened. The breath, trying to form words, tells us the child is upset: "Mo . . . Mommy! Hahuha (hic) ahhh hahu (sob)!!!"

"Sweetie, I can see you are very upset, but I can't understand what you're saying. Please calm down and tell me what happened."

Meanwhile, *your* breath has become irregular as visions of a horrible incident fill your wild imagination. You want to be able to calm your child, but how? Embracing her, you softly kiss her fore-head and say, "Sweetie, take a deep breath. Now let it out slowly. Again. Good. Now, can you tell me what happened?" Her words can now be understood because her breath is in harmony with her thoughts and emotions. Fortunately, the crisis was not as monu-mental as you had imagined it to be. (It rarely is!)

What you were witnessing and experiencing was the child's breath mimicking the pattern of her thoughts and emotions. The mind picks up the erratic flow of breath and begins to get more excited, unaware that the mind itself was the cause of this irregu-larity. This then causes the breath to become more erratic, thus causing a cycle that is difficult to interrupt. The child was trying to tell you what happened, but she couldn't because her breath, guided by the mind and emotions, was too disturbed.

The traumas of childhood have become everyday occurrences in adulthood. Our thoughts and emotions may be just as chaotic and upset, but we have learned ways to keep the stressful thoughts and feelings trapped inside, and from that a greater disharmony manifests.

Next time you find yourself agitated by daily irritants, notice your breath. Chances are you are taking in a breath, holding it, and then letting it out quickly. Take a moment and adjust the pattern—have your breath flow in and out without hesitation or strain. The more upset you are, the more difficult this will seem. Stay with it for a minute or longer, and you will be amazed how the thoughts and feelings respond.

*The universal life force* (prana) *is enhanced and guided through the harmonious rhythm of the breath* (Pranayama).

*The movement of the life force is influenced by inhalation, exhalation, and sustained breath.*

II.51 *A balanced, rhythmic pattern steadies the mind and emotions, causing the breath to become motionless.*

II.52 *As a result, the veils over the inner light are lifted.*

II.53 *The vista of higher consciousness is revealed.*

*Pranayama's* physical and mental effects have the supreme purpose of leading us into the stillness necessary for meditation. It is a wonderful practice to be done immediately before meditation. *Asana* steadies the body; *Pranayama* aligns the mental and emotional patterns. We will then guide the senses through *Pratyahara,* allowing us to focus and dive deep within.

Through the continual practice of *Pranayama,* the breath will understand that its workload has been greatly reduced. As the inhalation and exhalation slow, their stillness initiates the phase of motionless breath. It is a very natural and comfortable state, unlike the strained holding of breath we witness when upset. With a deepening in meditation, the *prana,* mind, and emotions grow still, causing a spontaneous stoppage of the breath (*Kevala Kumbaka*). The *prana* moves inward, flowing through the *Shushumna* to merge with the energy stored in the spine (*Kundalini*), which then moves magnetically upward, propelling us to higher consciousness.

The practice of *Pranayama* slowly allows the veils covering our True Self to lift. We are able to ascend unencumbered toward the light and merge with our divine nature.

*A balanced, rhythmic pattern steadies the mind and emotions, causing the breath to become motionless.*

*As a result, the veils over the inner light are lifted.*

*The vista of higher consciousness is revealed.*

## EXPERIENCING A BALANCE OF THE *PINGALA* (MASCULINE) AND THE *IDA* (FEMININE) THROUGH ALTERNATE-NOSTRIL BREATHING

(Please note: This breathing practice allows us to utilize the full lung capacity, taking in approximately seven times the amount of oxygen as in our normal shallow breathing. The chest muscles and the lungs may not be accustomed to such expansion, so be extra alert to any strain or dizziness. If you begin to get tired or short of breath, return to normal breathing for a few breaths; and then, after resting, continue. This will help to build up your stamina without strain. Strain or stress actually depletes the life force, erasing many of the good effects from the breathing practice.)

*This breathing practice is done in a comfortable seated position. It is a great practice to do anytime to calm yourself, or as a wonderful gateway to meditation.*

*With the right hand, make a gentle fist and release the thumb, the ring finger, and the little finger. This is a classic hand position in Yoga called* Vishnu mudra *(sustaining seal). If it is uncomfortable, you can use the thumb and index finger. The thumb gently presses the right nostril closed while the left nostril remains open. Then the extended fingers gently close the left nostril and the thumb releases the right nostril. (The left hand is resting comfortably on the lap.)*

To begin, exhale fully through both nostrils. Close off the right nostril with your thumb and inhale slowly through the left nostril as you expand the belly and the lower lungs. Continue to inhale to the upper chest. Feel the collarbones rise slightly.

Close off the left nostril with the fingers and exhale through the right nostril, releasing the air from the upper chest, the lower chest, and the abdomen—one section flowing into the other.

Inhale through the right nostril, expanding the abdomen and lower chest, the middle chest, and the upper chest, so that the collarbones rise slightly. Close off the right nostril with the thumb and exhale through the left nostril.

Continue this pattern. Exhale, inhale, switch nostrils; exhale, inhale, switch. Begin to practice for one minute and gradually increase up to three minutes or longer.

At the end of three minutes, as you come around to the right nostril, end with an exhalation. Allow the hand to come to the lap. Be still for a few moments with the eyes closed as you observe how calm and still the breath and mind have become. Observe the relationship between the two.

II.54 *Encouraging the senses to draw inward is* Pratyahara.

## ii.55 *Glimpsing the inner light, the senses contentedly dwell within.*

*Pratyahara* is the subtlest aspect of *Hatha Yoga*. It is a prelude to meditation. Most meditation techniques begin by enticing the senses to draw inward, allowing the mind to follow.

The five senses (*manas*), encouraged by curiosity (*ahamkara*), link up with the intellect (*buddhi*) and coax us outward from our inner consciousness. Even before birth, the senses feed us enormous amounts of information for both survival and enjoyment. With time, if we engage exclusively in the outer sphere of the senses, our inner world is forgotten.

Incredibly powerful, our senses expose us to the infinite spectrum of the universe. For thousands of years we have been awed and humbled by the sun, the moon, and the night sky. By developing highly refined instruments, we observe the far reaches of the universe, which are merely the portals to the multitude of undiscovered worlds millions of light-years away.

Venturing outward into the cosmic universe has triggered a polarity that draws us deeper within, creating a passion for the miraculous workings of the human body. Traveling inward with the help of technology, we explore atoms, DNA strands, and subatomic particles that we have yet to meet. Persistent in investigating both frontiers, we hope to learn the secrets to our existence.

With spiritual maturity, our inward explorations go beyond the physical world to explore the mystical fields. This necessitates a relaxation on the grasp our outer senses have on the external world. Because of the degree of overstimulation (*Rajas*) in our modern society, this can be a difficult shift. Accustomed to going every which way they please, the senses need to be cajoled as they rotate inward toward this new journey. If this overstimulation prevails on the inward focus, it stirs agitation and disharmony in our mind and emotions. This is why at the onset of inward practice, some report that they feel *less peaceful* than before. But with continuous guidance from the *Yamas* and *Niyamas,* the senses grow calm.

***Encouraging the senses to draw inward is* Pratyahara.**

***Glimpsing the inner light, the senses contentedly dwell within.***

## THE BEAUTY OF THE SUBTLE WORLDS DRAWS US INWARD

Gently enticing the senses to draw within often starts with our strongest information gatherer: the power of sight. More than 75 percent of information gathered from the external world is assembled from what we *see*.

Redirecting the seeing to an internal focus encourages all the other senses to follow. Because we load so many visual images in our minds, we continue to "see" even with the eyes closed. Often students learning to meditate are coached to establish their inward gaze between the eyebrows (to their "third eye") or at the heart center. With this slow and gentle training, the mind will gradually relinquish its projection of previously imprinted visual images.

Carefully choosing our outward images can help the inner vision to calm. Watching a visually frightening movie encourages the reflection of the same forces in our innermost worlds. At times it might be difficult to know if the images have staked a temporary or permanent residency within your mind. For a deeper level of practice, you may choose to withdraw, even temporarily, to a simple place in nature that affords very little outward stimulation.

As the "sight" firmly adheres to the inner world, the sense of hearing follows. Refining the level and quality of sound we regularly experience prepares us for the subtle internal sounds. The innermost melodies are orchestrated by the *prana* as it travels through the subtle nerve channels (*nadis*). We become captivated by a delicate hum or swish as it transforms into the celestial sound of bells, whispers, and choirs of angels.

## DEVELOPING EXTRAORDINARY SENSES

The subtler senses of touch, smell, and taste join seeing and hearing in their quest for inner vistas. As the senses find comfort in their inward journey, the "ordinary" senses become refined and powerful. We have tapped into the subtle realm of "extrasensory perception." What we then "see" is not physical. We "hear" what has not yet been said, "smell" what is not apparent, "feel" what we know to be true. These are some of the extraordinary powers described in the *Yoga Sutras* in book III, "*Vibhuti Pada:* The Divine Manifestation of Power," as the fruits of spiritual practice.

A mother can often "see" what her child is doing even if the child is out of "normal" sight. Sometimes mothers are said to have eyes in the backs of their heads because they "see" beyond the normal scope of vision.

Moments before her death, Saint Thérèse of Lisieux, known as the Little Flower, saw a vision of Mother Mary surrounded by hundreds of roses. Although those present in the room could not *see* this vision, the overwhelming fragrance of roses permeated the room. From that day forward, anyone who prayed to Saint Thérèse knew their prayers were heard when the unmistakable *scent of roses* enveloped the room.

*Encouraging the senses to draw inward is* Pratyahara.

*Glimpsing the inner light, the senses contentedly dwell within.*

Often we learn of situations in which someone was warned of impending danger by a voice not connected to a physical body.

I experienced such a lifesaving voice while camping by a lazy river in the Colorado mountains. Having pitched the tent and eaten to our appetites' fill, it was time to snuggle into our sleeping bags and be lulled to sleep by the sounds of nature. A river's voice can be the perfect lullaby.

Not remembering drifting off to sleep, I was suddenly and quite rudely awakened by a voice. Loud and clear it said, "Get up right now, pull up your tent, collect all your gear, and head for higher ground."

I peeked outside, and the moon's reflection on the water told my "regular" senses that everything was as it should be. But why did this voice wake me with such a message? Trusting that I had been given this warning for a reason, I timidly woke my tentmate.

More than a bit annoyed, she acquiesced to my emphatic rendition of the "higher" communication that I had heard. We pulled up camp and spent the rest of the night restlessly sleeping in our car in front of a restaurant that was closed for the night.

The next morning dawned clear and bright, and I was ready to concede defeat, accepting all the teasing I surely deserved. Eating breakfast in the restaurant, we overheard the other patrons talking with great concern about how last night the river had risen and flooded out the banks. "Sure hope no one was camping there," I heard several people say, as I said silent prayers of gratitude—not only that I had been warned but also that I had listened!

Once asked by a keen student how she could develop her extrasensory perception, Sri Swami Satchidanandaji smiled and said, "Why would you want to take on *extra* when you have difficulty handling the ordinary senses you have now? If you invite these extra-powerful senses, make sure you are strong enough to handle them."

The external world will fail to amuse the senses as you create an extraordinary world within. Entice the senses inward by invoking a gentle light or flame, the sound of your heartbeat, the fragrance of roses, the sweetness of saliva, or a feeling of well-being. Find ways to see, hear, and feel beauty in the delicate world within. As the outward senses are calm, meditation becomes effortless.

*Encouraging the senses to draw inward is* Pratyahara.

*Glimpsing the inner light, the senses contentedly dwell within.*

### EXPERIENCING THE SENSES AND AWARENESS DRAWING INWARD

*This is a profound relaxation practice for bringing in all of the outward sensual consciousness. We begin with the physical body, then move to the breath, thoughts, and emotions.*

*Begin to take in a few deep breaths. Notice how still the body and breath become as they relax. Observe the breath without controlling it as it comes and goes without any strain.*

*Guide this gentle breath to bring all sensual awareness from the feet, ankles, lower legs, knees, thighs, hips. Relax.*

*Guide this awareness to withdraw from the fingers, hands, wrists, forearms, elbows, upper arms.*

*Let go of holding awareness in the hands and arms or shoulders. Relax.*

*Do the same with the buttocks and pelvis, allow the abdomen to soften, and imagine the chest, lungs, heart, and throat relaxed.*

*Gently allow the awareness from the base of the spine to slowly rise up through the middle spine to the upper spine. Relax the shoulders and allow the neck to be an open connection between the heart and the head. Relax.*

*Experience the sensations as the body retreats.*

*The head holds most of the organs of the senses. Gently relax the jaw and withdraw taste and speech from the mouth.*

*Withdraw smell from the nose.*

*Allow the eyelids and the eyes to soften, moving toward the inner sight.*

*Relax the forehead, and tune the ears to the inner sounds. Relax the entire scalp and bathe the brain with relaxation.*

*Allow the gentle breath to relieve the mind and emotions of all movement. Relax.*

*Slowly bring the awareness to the gentle breath as it enters and leaves the body.*

*As it enters, feel yourself drawing deeper within.*

*As it leaves, feel yourself letting go of all holdings.*

*Notice a lightness and a feeling of distancing from the body, mind, emotions, and all worldly cares.*

*Begin to go further within to look for that place of stillness, peace, and joy. This is the dwelling place of your Divine Self.*

*(Have five full minutes of quiet time.)*

*Slowly and gently bring the awareness back to the breath.*

*Begin to increase the inhalation and feel that the senses have been purified and strengthened. Begin to feel them awakening to a relaxed body and a calm mind.*

*As you continue with this practice, your senses will become accustomed to drawing inward. It will become effortless to prepare the mind and emotions for deeper practice.*

# PART II

# FROM DEVOTED PRACTICE
# TO HIGHER CONSCIOUSNESS

BOOK III

# VIBHUTI PADA

*The Divine Manifestation of Power*

&

BOOK IV

# KAIVALYA PADA

*Supreme Liberation*

*Venturing into books III and IV, we find ourselves introduced to*
*a different type of learning. The earlier padas implied that as we*
*become more adept at the practices, the secrets of Yoga will be*
*revealed. You may already be reaping these benefits and insights.*
*Even during our exploration of books III and IV, we will continue to*
*reference books I and II, as they are the basis of spiritual practice.*

*Until now, the more subtle teachings may have eluded you. They*
*might have seemed superfluous or unrelatable to your life and*
*practices. When the plethora of knowledge revealed in the sutras has*
*expanded your mind and heart, the yearning for further study*
*is present.*

*It is important, as we delve into mystical and subtle realms, to*
*remember that concepts are best assimilated when the deeper*
*spiritual practices are regular and steady. Books III and IV*
*incorporate the energy generated from our dedicated practices to*
*propel us into subtle states of being.*

*Both* Vibhuti Pada *and* Kaivalya Pada *describe psychic and spiritual*
*powers* (siddhis) *as the fruits gained through spiritual practice.*
*Although the attainment of these powers can be a way of evaluating*
*spiritual progress, we are well and strongly advised not to dwell on*
*them, as they detract us from the ultimate realization of*
*the Divine Self.*

*The irony is that* Vibhuti Pada *has the greatest number of sutras of all the* padas! *Also, the explanation of the* siddhis *continues into book IV. It is a bit like describing the tasty treats in the cookie jar to a six-year-old while expounding upon the unhealthy effects of sugar, white flour, and butter. It would be as difficult to convince the Yoga student not to hope for the powers as it would be to keep those little fingers out of the cookie jar.*

*Book III begins with the last three sutras of the Eight-Faceted Path* (Asthaanga Yoga): Dharana *(contemplation),* Dhyana *(meditation), and* Samadhi *(union with the Divine Self). These final three facets are more internal than the preceding five, and as they flow seamlessly one into the other, it is known as* Samyama *(fusion). With* Samyama *comes knowledge of the Divine Self. Accompanying this realization is the manifestation* (Vibhuti) *of psychic and spiritual powers* (siddhis). *The culmination of book III describes the myriad powers born of* Samyama, *the fusion of* Dharana, Dhyana, *and* Samadhi.

*While both* Vibhuti Pada *and* Kaivalya Pada *describe the* siddhis, *it is in book IV that we understand the depth of understanding necessary to merge with the Divine Self, leaving the tantalizing* siddhis *behind.*

*If you venture regularly into the* subtler *aspects of Yoga, the psychic powers are certain to beckon to you. While they can be entertaining*

*and interesting, they are not worthy of our complete dedication,
since they distract from the superior illumination and peace beyond
their horizons. They may initially excite us, because we have not
encountered them before. We would be just as amazed watching
TV for the first time—all those little people moving about in that
tiny box. In that way the ordinary mind becomes dazzled by the
display of yogic powers. The yogis in their equanimity recognize all
these powers as natural aspects of the expanded mind and emotions.
If they are naturally revealed to you, use this precious gift for the
greater good.*

*These experiences may visit us during our formal practices or at any
other time. We may see flashing lights or angels, hear the phone
before it rings, choose the scenic road only to find out later that
the main highway had been closed for repair, smell blossoms in the
winter, or in any number of other ways encounter the extraordinary.*

*Often a disciple may be enticed by these powers (siddhis). It is then
the role of a guru or spiritual teacher to guide and keep the disciple
out of harm's way.*

*This is the story of one disciple's experience: The long-awaited
day of her annual interview with the guru caused her to become
very excited. Each year since she came to the ashram, the teacher
had asked the same question: "How are you progressing with your
meditation?" The disciple each time had no choice but to give the*

*same answer: "I am not able to focus my mind and heart for even*
*one moment."*

But this time she had some wonderful experiences to share. She
began by telling the guru about the bright lights shooting from the
base of her spine, often accompanied by loud chiming sounds. She
watched as her beloved teacher carefully listened to her extolling her
experiences. As the disciple waited with bated breath to be praised
and told how she was finally accelerating rapidly in her spiritual
growth, the clever guru did the unexpected. Leaning over, the
sage touched her on the top of her head, uttering the words "Don't
worry, this will never happen again." And it never did. As the wise
Paramahansa Yogananda said, "Meditation is not a circus. Do not be
caught by the bright lights and sounds."

*Allow yourself to be totally dedicated to the ultimate realization: the*
*knowledge of your Divine Self.*

# VIBHUTI PADA

## The Divine Manifestation of Power

*Entering "Vibhuti Pada: The Divine Manifestation of Power," it always intrigues me that only five of the eight facets of Asthaanga Yoga have commentaries in book II, "Sadhana Pada: Cultivation of Spiritual Practice." The last three, Dharana (contemplation), Dhyana (meditation), and Samadhi (union with the Divine), are allocated to book III, Vibhuti Pada. It affirms that they are not practices in themselves; rather, they are progressive internal states that evolve from the earlier cultivated practices. Opening the doors to the Divine Manifestation of Power, "doing" transforms into "being."*

# ANTARA YOGA:
## The Inner Quest

W HEN THE FIVE preceding facets of *Asthaanga* have been effectively interwoven, we are gifted with *Antara Yoga*, the inner quest. With continued devotion, *Dharana* (contemplation) and *Dhyana* (meditation) guide us to the innermost treasure, *Samadhi* (union with Divine Consciousness). When they seamlessly flow from one to another, it is known as *Samyama* (fusion).

*Gathering consciousness and focusing it within is* Dharana *(contemplation).*

*The continuous inward flow of consciousness is* Dhyana *(meditation).*

*When individual consciousness unites with the Divine Consciousness, the illusion of separateness dissolves; this is* Samadhi.

*When* Dharana *(contemplation),* Dhyana *(meditation), and* Samadhi *(union with Divine Consciousness) seamlessly merge into one another, this is* Samyama *(fusion).*

*Through* Samyama, *individual and Divine Consciousness gracefully reunite.*

## III.1 *Gathering consciousness and focusing it within is* Dharana *(contemplation).*

If we are well primed, the transition to these subtle levels from the other preceding practices is effortless. Many may choose to "do meditation," but this is more often than not a technique derived from *Pratyahara* practice (encouraging the senses inward).

Following the flow of *Yamas* and *Niyamas* as the first two facets of *Asthaanga Yoga,* we know that, as we develop reverence and devotion for others and ourselves, the mind and emotions become tranquil. *Asana* and *Pranayama,* the third and fourth facets, allow the life force to gather and refine, bringing ease to the body, mind, and emotions. Then *Pratyahara,* the fifth facet, encourages the senses inward. Each of the facets, when practiced with dedication and respect, naturally leads us to the threshold of the Divine Manifestation of Power. It is a progression that can be neither quickened nor affected.

Observing the potential beauty of a rosebud, we may be eager to see it in full bloom. Becoming impatient with the process and taking nature into our own hands, if we peel the petals, hoping to create a full bloom, it would destroy both the sweet bud and the exquisite blossom. Maturity cannot be forced; it takes time, patience, and nurturing. Nature is a great teacher, showing us that everything develops at the perfect time.

The three graduated stages that are presented in these sutras are meant to exhibit a quantitative rather than qualitative difference. The same attention and awareness that are present in *Dharana* (contemplation) are also brought to *Dhyana* (meditation) and the lower states of *Samadhi* (union with Divine Consciousness). The different phases are determined by the length of time our consciousness is able to remain engaged within.

Imagine this process similarly to applying oil to a tough piece of leather so that it may become supple. The length of time the oil is allowed to remain on the leather is crucial to the process. For it to soak in and soften the leather, it is best to leave it on for a long time. If the oil is applied and then removed within twenty seconds, the softening effect is minimal. If it stays for two minutes, the absorption process is able to begin. When the oil remains on the leather for half an hour or longer, it is completely absorbed, leaving the leather pliable and without a residue.

This is similar to the way *Dharana* (contemplation), *Dhyana* (meditation), and *Samadhi* (union with Divine Consciousness) respectively affect the realization of our Divine Self. As we are able to gather our awareness and engage it within for a short amount of time, we are experiencing *Dharana*. If we engage it for a longer time, we experience *Dhyana*. Yet more time allows for total absorption, *Samadhi*.

## AN EASEFUL AWARENESS

*Dharana* is most commonly translated as "concentration" and is frequently used synonymously and interchangeably with the word "meditation." Defining it as "concentration" suggests an intense focusing of the mind. This characterization can cause our bodies to tense and our breathing to become irregular, and while our senses are alerted to the mission at hand, there is little comfort or ease. More accurately, *Dharana* invites us into an easeful awareness that prompts the flow of consciousness back to its source. In choosing an English equivalent for *Dharana*, "contemplation" or "reflection" is more in keeping with the effect we want to evoke.

Through *Dharana*, our thoughts, feelings, and actions interweave, inducing a pattern of consciousness that flows harmoniously to the source.

*Gathering consciousness and focusing it within is* Dharana
*(contemplation).*

## HARMONIZE WITH YOUR TRUE VIBRATION

In book I, sutras 34–39, we are offered a selection of uplifting
ways to lead the mind and emotions to *Dharana* and *Dhyana.* The
sutras, being very empowering and nonrestrictive, after offering us
many choices, ultimately leave the path open-ended. For example,
I.39: *Or dedicate yourself to anything that elevates and embraces your
heart.* These two simple criteria for selecting a focus, elevation and
embracing, seem agreeable to most anyone.

The first part of sutra I.39 suggests that the focus be both uplifting
*and* inspiring. This gives you the freedom to choose almost anything
you wish: a chakra or a spiritual center on the body, a great and
inspiring being, a prayer or a sacred word; the options are infinite.
Choose carefully, so that the qualities held within the sacred object
will have the power to escort you to the depth of your Divine Self.

The second suggestion is that you love it, and that it elevates you
to a state of joy. When you select something you love, your heart
will want to embrace it fully.

Many of us have experienced elevating feelings from being in
love. At those times our complete awareness is funneled into one
special person—all of our senses and thoughts are with them; just
to think about them uplifts us and brings joy.

Imagine you're at an airport waiting for your sweetheart. While
standing there waiting for the aircraft to come in, your feet may
hurt a bit, or hunger may remind you that in your haste you for-
got to eat. But the moment you see your beloved, energy suddenly
floods your body, leaping out through your heart and rushing to
embrace her or him. Your aching feet and hunger are forgotten.
The experience of contemplation is usually not quite as visceral or

dramatic. Yet if we truly love what we are focusing on, with time and practice, the energy flows to the centers of higher consciousness, propelled by our devotion. We are filled with joy and bliss.

Even if you are given a focus for practice by a teacher, or learn one from a tried-and-true tradition, it is important to adapt it as you embrace it with your whole heart.

A friend of mine, who had a long career as a cardiac surgeon, went on a ten-day meditation retreat. When he returned, I asked him how the experience had been for him. "Oh, it was fine," he answered, still somewhat preoccupied. "Tell me something. They told us to meditate on the *hara* [an energy center used in the Buddhist tradition]. I spent the whole time trying to figure out exactly where it was. Dusting off my memory, I went through my old *Gray's Anatomy* book from medical school, but I couldn't find the *hara*. I kept wondering if it was to the left or right, above or below the pancreas. Can you help clarify it for me?"

Chuckling to myself and at the same time appreciating his dilemma, I said, "Let's make this easy. Do you know where your heart is?"

"Of course I know where my heart is—and everybody else's, too," answered the experienced surgeon.

"Put your full and complete attention at the heart center and all the love that flows through it. That seems to be a perfect focus for you!" I said. He looked relieved as a smile appeared in his sparkling eyes.

In this case my friend was offered a focus that was not in harmony with his vibration. When you settle on something suited to you, become completely devoted to it. Sometimes after a while we become impatient, thinking, "Oh, this technique is not working for me." We may then read a book or hear a teacher proclaim a "better way" and decide to try that approach. By switching techniques, you will not reach the depth or steadiness that you need to find your true center.

## GO DEEP

There's a popular adage about digging shallow wells: If you dig down ten feet in one well and hit rock and then move to another place and dig down ten feet to no avail and then move again, you may never get water. But if you continue to dig deeper in one well—thirty, forty feet—eventually you will be rewarded.

If you spend your energy continually digging shallow wells, you will not know where to go to find refuge when something happens during the day to upset your equilibrium. Being faithful to one method, you can dive deep into that safe haven and merge with the inner stillness.

You may feel you are still "playing the field" with a variety of techniques. Gradually begin to embrace *one* closest to your temperament, and "date" only that one for a while. After a few weeks, you might get "engaged" to it, or you may decide it is not for you. Then select another. Stay with that one for a month or so. After two or three tries, choose *one,* make your "marriage" plans, and be faithful to your choice. Apply wholehearted devotion and let it escort you to your own heart, deep within.

**Gathering consciousness and focusing it within is** Dharana **(contemplation).**

### EXPERIENCING CONTEMPLATION (*DHARANA*) THROUGH *TRADAKA*, OR GAZING

(Please note: This practice is a wonderful example of *Pratyahara* flowing into *Dharana*. It begins with an external physical focus and then draws you inward to the subtle image. It then alternates both an outward and inward focus, coordinating the eyes with the mind and emotions so they function as one. The outward gaze toward the external object is "seen," when we close our eyes, by our inner vision. As the internal image dims, we again open our eyes and gaze outward to the physical form of the image. The practice is continued until our consciousness gathers and is persuaded to remain inward as *Dharana* [contemplation].)

*Choose an inspirational object: a lit candle, a photo, flowers, the sunrise or sunset, a mandala or yantra (which is a sacred geometric pattern), or anything that uplifts and evokes a quiet, peaceful feeling.*

*Sit directly in front of it so it is at eye level, close enough for you to see the form and feel its qualities.*

*(Because it is not necessary to distinguish details, glasses or contact lenses may be removed, permitting the eyes to relax and soften.)*

*Close your eyes. Take in a few deep breaths and let them out slowly as your body stills.*

*Slowly open the eyes halfway. Begin to gaze at your chosen object; the eyes and eyelids remain relaxed and soft.*

*Resist the temptation to reach out and grasp the image with your vision; instead, keep the eyes soft; allow the image to flow toward you.*

*At first, the eyes may wander. Gently bring them back to the chosen object. The breath continues to be gentle.*

*Allow the eyes to be directed outward until they blink, tear, or feel any discomfort. Then close them softly.*

*Observe the image as it now appears in the mind's eye. Gently perceive the same inspirational qualities as you go deep within.*

*When the inner image begins to fade, open the eyes again and gaze toward the external object.*

*If the mind starts to wander and brings in stories about the object or something totally unrelated, gently bring your awareness back to the object in front of you.*

*Repeat this sequence several times, gazing outward and gazing inward.*

*Let all thoughts and feelings drift into the background as you contemplate your sacred object.*

*If any tension creeps into the body, take in a few deep breaths and let it go.*

*After a few minutes, allow the eyes to close, drawing deep within. Clearly "see" the image with the inner eye. Be silent for a few minutes and enjoy the inner stillness of* Dharana.

## III.2 *The continuous inward flow of consciousness is* Dhyana *(meditation)*.

With continued inward awareness, *Dharana* (contemplation) transports us into *Dhyana* (meditation).

In *Dharana* (contemplation), the length of time consciousness dwells with the Divine is limited to a few seconds, causing the sense of peace we derive from *Dharana* to be transient. In *Dhyana* (meditation), the gathered consciousness nestles more comfortably into our divine essence.

The distinction between the two stages is similar to the action of oil (awareness) being poured from a small vessel (*chitta*) back into the infinite sea (*chit*). *Dharana* intermittently touches inner awareness, similar to the way oil pours from a full cylinder, stopping ever so briefly before the next plop follows. There is a definite start and end to the periods of inner awareness, and often they happen so quickly that we miss the inner experience.

Because of these frequent fluctuations in the state of *Dharana,* our awareness vacillates from the external to the internal, between "doing" and "being," back and forth. *Dhyana* (meditation) is analogous to the oil (awareness) flowing in a *continuous* stream from the small vessel (*chitta*) back to the infinite sea (*chit*) of consciousness. With *Dhyana,* the awareness remains within for a longer time. This allows our identification with the Divine to increase. Even when the "formal" meditation is completed, a part of us is always rooted within. *Dhyana* propels our consciousness toward the vast sea of the Divine. Less determined thoughts and emotions are coaxed to flow with it toward the source. This dynamic experience of meditation brims over, touching every aspect of life. The aura (*pranic* body) becomes luminous with this dynamic power, giving you a magnetic and vibrant personality. As this power continues to deepen, people are drawn to you and are affected by your cheerfulness, your immeasurable energy, and your joy. Your peace and strength are elevated by the boundless source that you have accessed. The unpleasant situations that you once avoided are now understood, and in some cases welcomed. You are able to observe that all things have a greater purpose, even if that purpose is sometimes hidden. People you once experienced as foreign or strange can be embraced by your open and loving heart. A whole new perspective has unfolded.

**The continuous inward flow of consciousness is Dhyana (meditation).**

You may find it necessary to withdraw from the world for a time to continue nourishing this dynamic power. Or, as is often the case with this newfound energy, you may find yourself inspired to serve others and yourself with greater zeal.

The state of *Dhyana* expands our understanding of the world around us, and of ourselves. We are able to delight in the newfound bliss that up to this time had been held in reserve. In *Dhyana* we transcend the physical, mental, and emotional realms, and we experience infinite joy.

**The continuous inward flow of consciousness is Dhyana (meditation).**

## EXPERIENCING THE MEDITATIVE STATE
### (*DHYANA*)

*Sit in a comfortable position, relax the body and breath, and allow the senses to draw inward. Focus the awareness on the place between the eyebrows, the third eye.*

*As you become still, observe the sound of the breath as it enters the body and whispers the sound "so." Listen to the breath as it leaves. "Hum." "So-hum. So-hum."*

*Join the breath by silently repeating "so" with the inhalation. Silently repeat "hum" with the exhalation. (This is* japa, *repetition of a mantra.)*

*"So-hum," "So-hum," "So-hum." (This invokes the vibration of "I am.")*

*Listen to the whisper of the rhythm of life as it flows in and out of the body. It is affirming both nature ("so") and spirit ("hum"). Recognizing both parts of us in harmony, it calls us to the light within.*

*"So-hum." "So-hum." "So-hum." "So-hum." "So-hum." "So-hum." "So-hum."*

*Continue listening as you softly repeat this mantra for ten minutes or longer.*

*After a time allow the "so-hum" mantra to repeat itself (ajapa). "So-hum" will take you to the place where the body, mind, and breath dissolve into the Divine.*

### III.3 *When individual consciousness unites with the Divine Consciousness, the illusion of separateness dissolves; this is* Samadhi.

The world that we visit during *Samadhi* (union with Divine Consciousness) has no tangible language. It is a state beyond description. It can only be experienced.

If we stir a cup of sugar into a pitcher of water, it *seems* to disappear. We may not be able to *see* it, yet if we *taste* the water, we recognize the sugar by its sweetness. Because the sugar has been completely absorbed in the water, their union creates a new expression. From then on it becomes impossible to separate the two.

The effect of the sugar merging with the water is similar to our gathered consciousness merging into the Divine. When consciousness unites in *Samadhi,* unlike during *Dharana* (contemplation) or *Dhyana* (meditation), the distinction between the individual consciousness (*chitta*) and the eternal consciousness (*chit*) dissolves.

Trying to comprehend *Samadhi* (union with Divine Consciousness) before we have experienced it is like trying to understand being in love before it happens. A child might ask her mother what it feels like to be in love. With great introspection, her mother may answer, "It is not something that can be explained in words. It is beyond our understanding of what joy can mean. All I can say is you will know it when it happens!" *Samadhi* is like that.

The different stages and degrees of *Samadhi* (union with Divine Consciousness) are described and defined in book I, chapter 7, sutras 40–51. As we might remember, some of these elevated states are temporary (*Sabija*); they still hold seeds that can sprout. These states, while very powerful, are not potent enough to eliminate all the seeds of karma. Even if it *appears* that our minds and emotions have been totally transformed, the seeds have the ability to germinate given the proper conditions. We may attain those grand heights for a time and then be relegated back to the jurisdiction of the mind and emotions.

*When individual consciousness unites with the Divine Consciousness, the illusion of separateness dissolves; this is* **Samadhi.**


## HIDING ANGER IN A CAVE

There is a wonderful story of a woman who was burdened with a terrible temper. Everything ignited this anger. To control this problem, she decided to retreat into a cave for deep spiritual practice. After spending ten years without seeing another human being, she was convinced the anger had been conquered.

When she finally emerged from the cave and was about to once again enter the world, a crowd gathered, drawn by her vibrant spiritual power. They had known her before and were curious to observe the change.

"What was it like?" one person in the crowd asked. "Did you get angry at all?" said another.

"For the entire time, not once did I get angry," she proudly reported.

"It is difficult for me to believe that with the degree of anger you had when you went in, you did not get angry even once," a woman chided.

"No, not even *once.*" The cave dweller kept to her story.

"Do you mean that even if a wild animal came up to your cave and disturbed your meditation, you did not get angry? I really cannot accept what you say as truth," said the same woman, continuing to pursue the issue.

"Listen, *you fool,* I told you, NOTHING DISTURBED MY PEACE AND I NEVER GOT ANGRY. Now leave me alone!"

If the seeds are still fertile, they are always available to sprout. In the deeper states of *Samadhi,* consciousness forever rests in unity with the Divine; then not even a seed is left to germinate.

When one exists in this exalted state, all former identities—woman, man, doctor, nurse, mother, father, Jewish, Christian, Hindu, Muslim—dissolve into oneness. While we still care for and appreciate the body, mind, and emotions as vehicles for living in this physical world, our identification with them lessens. We then may lose interest in anything to do with the physical world, including food, clothing, shelter, and even our relationships. Only a hair-breadth thread tethers us to our earthly existence.

Our identity has merged with our divine nature, the all-pervading light within. *Samadhi,* as described by the saints and sages, is a completely different realm of reality from that of our everyday experiences.

We are often inspired by the consciousness brought forth in *Samadhi* to serve the world from that rich understanding. Once we have been ignited by Divine Consciousness, our view of service is forever transformed. With purity of heart and mind, our spiritual vibrations travel through an infinite distance, infusing peace to thousands. We act now out of the knowledge of oneness.

Whichever level of *Samadhi* is experienced, our previous way of understanding life is forever changed. Once we embrace the Divine, our memory clears, as we know who we are without doubt or question. We have fallen in love with our Divine Self.

*When individual consciousness unites with the Divine Consciousness, the illusion of separateness dissolves; this is* **Samadhi.**

## EXPERIENCING THE FLOW OF *DHARANA* (CONTEMPLATION), *DHYANA* (MEDITATION), AND *SAMADHI* (UNION WITH DIVINE CONSCIOUSNESS)

(Please note: This experience is presented to help clarify the evolution and relationship of *Dharana* [contemplation], *Dhyana* [meditation], and *Samadhi* [union with Divine Consciousness]. As mentioned earlier, these are not practices in themselves; rather, they are progressive internal "states" that evolve through the influence of conscious living and the other practices that preceded them. If these states are invoked by transforming the effort of "doing" into the natural ease of "being," grace is bestowed.)

*Assume a comfortable and relaxed sitting position. Have the base of the spine directed toward the earth, while the top of the head reaches in the direction of the heavens.*

*Choose an inspirational object for* Dharana *(contemplation), something or someone your heart embraces. It could be your sweetheart, child, parent, or friend, or anything that embodies the essence of divinity for you, such as a statue, picture, or photo. It is effective as long as it uplifts you and allows for an all-encompassing pathway to love.*

*Begin to inwardly or outwardly observe all the qualities your senses can elicit.*

*What are you seeing? Beauty, grace, colors, tones, shapes?*

*What are you touching? Is it soft, smooth, rounded, sensual, solid?*

*What are you hearing? Is it gentle, strong, inviting, mesmerizing?*

*What fragrance is enticing you? Is it sweet, fresh, feminine, masculine, flowery, celestial?*

*Is your sense of taste involved, perhaps with a kiss?*

*When you feel the presence of the object of devotion, are you peaceful, happy, joyous, loving?*

*Allow the physical eyes to close, and begin to cuddle up to all the sensory experiences now residing deep within your mind and heart. Embrace the person or the divine object completely as you encircle it with a feeling of infinite love.*

*This experience will escort you to the state of* Dharana *(contemplation).*

*If your heart forgets to embrace your beloved within, notice how your consciousness wanders away. At these times refresh your thoughts and feelings by either gazing outward or re-forming a clear image within, involving all the senses.*

*The state of* Dharana *(contemplation) holds only as long as you can stay present.*

*After a period of time (minutes, hours, days, weeks, maybe months or longer), the individual sensory perceptions begin to fade and become less defined. Then the identification with the object and its qualities recedes, and simultaneously a deep feeling of love emerges.*

Dharana *(contemplation)* has merged into Dhyana *(meditation)*.

With the immersion into Dhyana *(meditation)*, the cherished object reveals its essence: all-embracing love. With the unveiling of this knowledge, the indrawn focus becomes effortless.

Continue to dwell at this level of Dhyana *(meditation)* as the all-embracing love flourishes in your heart.

Now the threshold into Samadhi *(union with Divine Consciousness)* is easily traversed. Any remaining thoughts, feelings, and sensory perceptions of the external dissolve. Abounding love is your only experience.

With the immersion into Samadhi, your entire reality transforms. You experience this all-embracing love for everyone and everything.

III.4 *When* Dharana *(contemplation),* Dhyana *(meditation), and* Samadhi *(union with Divine Consciousness) seamlessly merge into one another, this is* Samyama *(fusion).*

## III.5 *Through* Samyama, *individual and Divine Consciousness gracefully reunite.*

*Samyama* (fusion) is the integration of *Dharana, Dhyana,* and *Samadhi. Samyama* starts with *Dharana* (contemplation), focusing on an objective. Here there is an awareness of an object separate from yourself. *Dharana* gracefully slides into *Dhyana* (meditation) when there is an unbroken flow of awareness, allowing identification with the divine essence of all things. Becoming completely immersed in that essence, individual consciousness merges with Divine Consciousness in *Samadhi* (union with Divine Consciousness).

In *Samyama* (fusion) the three aspects are perceived not as individual but as a single current flowing from uninterrupted awareness. This flow is seamless and without effort. Any effort immediately brings us back into the realm of thoughts and emotions. The ability to realize *Samyama* (fusion) may take years of devoted practice and purification.

*Samyama* is available in all aspects of life. From the spiritual to the scientific worlds, many great discoveries came through *Samyama.*

We can reflect on the story of the great Albert Einstein that we spoke about in sutra 1.43, when he experienced *Samadhi* on light. First he contemplated (*Dharana*) light, and with further awareness he was led into meditation (*Dhyana*) on light. These stages followed each other sequentially and united in *Samadhi.* With seamless merging, the experience became *Samyama.*

Einstein humbly proclaimed, "I did not discover light, I meditated on it [*Dhyana*], until it revealed itself to me [*Samadhi*]."

As these qualities expand with use, spreading them generously raises everyone's quality of life.

*When* Dharana *(contemplation),* Dhyana *(meditation), and* Samadhi *(union with Divine Consciousness) seamlessly merge into one another, this is* Samyama *(fusion).*

*Through* Samyama, *individual and Divine Consciousness gracefully reunite.*

# THE GIFTS OF *SAMYAMA*

CONTINUING OUR EXPLORATIOn of *Samyama*, we delve into the power the three subtle facets of *Asthaanga—Dharana, Dhyana,* and *Samadhi*—wield when they seamlessly merge. This union escorts us to the threshold of acquiring the notorious *siddhis.*

*The insights and wisdom gained through* Samyama *enhance all aspects of life.*

*The three facets that comprise* Samyama *(Dharana, Dhyana, and* Samadhi*) are more subtle than the preceding five.*

*Even these three facets that make up* Samyama *appear external when the seedless* Samadhi *(Nirbija) is experienced.*

*By observing the silent moments that occur between the rising thoughts and feelings without controlling them, consciousness is transformed and expanded (Nirodha Parinama).*

*As the transformation of consciousness (Nirodha Parinama) becomes steady, profound tranquility is experienced.*

*Then the fluctuations of consciousness are pacified, and
Samadhi (Samadhi Parinama) becomes a familiar state of
being.*

*From this all thoughts and feelings, without divergence, flow
into captivated awareness (Ekagrata Parinama).*

*Through the three phases of Samyama, the natural elements
are transformed, as are the thoughts, feelings, and senses,
securing and expanding the state of higher consciousness.*

III.6 *The insights and wisdom gained through* Samyama *enhance all aspects of life.*

The continuous flow of energy from *Dharana* to *Dhyana* transforms consciousness, placing us on the threshold of *Samadhi*. When the three are unified, their attributes merge, forming *Samyama,* the pathway to the *siddhis* and higher consciousness.

We are strongly cautioned not to leap over any of the stages, even as the mind tries to convince us that we are more advanced than we actually are. Adhering to this sequence ensures that great insights and wisdom are gained through continual practice. Therefore, all aspects of life expand, elevating our vision to the transcendental experience of the Divine Self.

**The insights and wisdom gained through** Samyama **enhance all aspects of life.**

III.7 *The three facets that comprise* Samyama (Dharana, Dhyana, *and* Samadhi) *are more subtle than the preceding five.*

Blending together in *Samyama,* the three subtle facets (*Dharana, Dhyana,* and *Samadhi*) create a dynamic energy, drawing us inward to meet the Divine Self encased in the heart.

The first five facets of *Asthaanga Yoga,* the Eight-Faceted Path, allows for balance of body, mind, and senses, which grants an easy transition to the inner worlds. The first two facets, *Yama* and *Niyama,* encourage us to refine and reflect our true nature. The third facet, *Asana,* concerns itself with the physical body, creating stillness and ease. The fourth facet, *Pranayama,* directs and enhances the life force. *Pratyahara,* the fifth facet, calms the senses and cajoles them inward.

These first five facets of *Asthaanga* require *action* to achieve their potential, while *Dharana, Dhyana,* and *Samadhi* display a more reflective state of being, engaged by the inner worlds.

**The three facets that comprise** Samyama (Dharana, Dhyana, **and** Samadhi) *are more subtle than the preceding five.*

## III.8 *Even these three facets that make up* Samyama *appear external when the seedless* Samadhi (Nirbija) *is experienced.*

With each step of evolutionary ascendance, we are aware of attaining a level of consciousness greater than the stage before. It can be equated with *seeing* light, *experiencing* light, and *being* light. The sequential experiences allow us to touch the source as we merge into the light.

Graced with *Nirbija Samadhi* (without seed), all aspects of *Dharana* and *Dhyana* appear external. This also applies to most of the *Samadhis* with seed, including *Sabija Samadhi.* These *Samadhis* allow us to taste the experience of merging with the Divine, but the bliss of this exalted state is only temporary. Until there is total absorption in *Nirbija Samadhi*, we are unable to realize complete and total union with the Divine Self.

**Even these three facets that make up** Samyama *appear external* **when the seedless** Samadhi (Nirbija) *is experienced.*

III.9 *By observing the silent moments that occur between the rising thoughts and feelings without controlling them, consciousness is transformed and expanded* (Nirodha Parinama).

Through careful observation we notice there is a pause between the rising thoughts and feelings. When immersed in *Dharana* or *Dhyana,* the duration between the moments expands and, if sustained, increases the experience of stillness. This observation leads us to *Nirodha Parinama,* where the chosen object loses its external captivation, trading it for a dynamic state of inner reflection.

In this way it is similar to the three aspects of breath: inhalation, exhalation, and retention. As we become adept at *Pranayama,* the interlude between the inhalation and exhalation and between the exhalation and inhalation becomes greater, causing a profound tranquility. When this occurs, the breath's integral connection with the mind causes elongated pauses between the movement of rising thoughts. It is in this profound stillness that consciousness expands and transforms.

*By observing the silent moments that occur between the rising thoughts and feelings without controlling them, consciousness is transformed and expanded* (Nirodha Parinama).

### EXPERIENCING THE SPACE
### BETWEEN THE BREATHS

*Find a comfortable seated position with the spine erect yet relaxed.*

*Take in a deep inhalation and retain the breath inward.*

*Notice how the space between the movements of the thoughts lengthens as the breath is being held.*

*Prolonging the moments between the breaths increases the moments of stillness.*

*Slowly and gently exhale, and pause as the breath ceases momentarily.*

*As you begin the next inhalation, notice if you can perceive an increase in the span of moments between the breaths.*

*Do they appear to lengthen? Is there more silence?*

*Inhale. Hold the breath. Observe the moments between thoughts.*

*Exhale. Hold. Observe.*

*Allow the breath to return to normal. Be still for a moment or longer.*

*The more the practice is done, the easier it becomes to merge into stillness.*

III.10 *As the transformation of consciousness* (Nirodha Parinama) *becomes steady, profound tranquility is experienced.*

When consciousness has transformed to such an extent that *any* external object is no longer subtle enough to be used for *Dharana* or *Dhyana,* consciousness itself becomes the focus. It gains the ability to calm its own fluctuations. This is done by observing the diminishing fluctuations of consciousness as it retreats into equanimity. The profound stillness then expands and extends through the borderless inner worlds. By placing the awareness *between* the movements, instead of, as is customary, being drawn into the movements, we find ourselves immersed in the sanctuary of serenity.

Often there is an urge, which even great teachers and texts encourage us to repress, to suppress or somehow inhibit "other" thoughts or feelings. Instead, if we place full awareness on our primary focus, the others will dissipate. If we try to focus on *not* doing something, it often takes more energy than the actual doing.

Observing two plants of similar size and vibrancy, if we begin to water and care for one, it will thrive. We do not need to do anything to destroy the other; benign neglect will suffice. The same applies to our thoughts and feelings: Nourish the ones we want to keep and let the others wither away.

**As the transformation of consciousness (Nirodha Parinama) becomes steady, profound tranquility is experienced.**

III.11 *Then the fluctuations of consciousness are pacified, and* Samadhi (Samadhi Parinama) *becomes a familiar state of being.*

III.12 *From this all thoughts and feelings, without divergence, flow into captivated awareness* (Ekagrata Parinama).

We have all experienced being captivated by a haunting melody, a radiant sunset, the smile of a small child. These sutras indicate that such experiences occur also on the subtle level as states of *Samadhi* are revealed. Instead of external objects riveting our attention, the magnificence of our true essence lures us inward. The inner sounds, sights, and feelings entice us, fading at the exact moment we merge with our Divine Self.

*Then the fluctuations of consciousness are pacified, and* Samadhi (Samadhi Parinama) *becomes a familiar state of being.*

*From this all thoughts and feelings, without divergence, flow into captivated awareness* (Ekagrata Parinama).

### EXPERIENCING CAPTIVATING AWARENESS

*(Please note: Although it is not possible to practice captivated awareness, this exercise can help to create a similar effect on ordinary thoughts and feelings. It is necessary to experience Samadhi before awareness can be fully captivated.)*

*Choose an external object that has a mesmerizing effect on the body, mind, emotions, and senses.*

*It could be the captivating vision of a sunset or sunrise. A haunting piece of music. The transporting fragrance of a flower. Any object that summons the extraordinary.*

*Begin to focus your total awareness on the chosen object.*

*Hold steady, allowing the vibration from the object to quiet the body and drift inward to calm the mind and emotions.*

*After a time, it will be difficult to distinguish the brilliance of the sunset or musical composition from your inner being.*

*You may feel an inward glow like the light from the sun as it rises or sets, or each cell may begin to vibrate to the inspiring piece of music.*

*Stay in that presence for as long as you are able.*

*When you feel ready, take in a few deep breaths, slowly open the eyes, and become present.*

*Allow the sublime vibration to continue even as you go about your day.*

*Repeat the practice often to activate that part of consciousness that yearns for oneness.*

III.13 *Through the three phases of* Samyama, *the natural elements are transformed, as are the thoughts, feelings, and senses, securing and expanding the state of higher consciousness.*

The natural progression of *Samyama* leads us to a permanent state of higher consciousness. As that becomes our reality, it supersedes all sensations, whether of body, mind, emotions, or the natural elements. This encourages us to dwell eternally in the peace of our divine nature.

When beginning a meditation practice, the first step is to choose an object conducive to meditation that is uplifting and touches our hearts. At the outset we are well advised to place our full awareness on that chosen object. But due to the lack of focus in the initial stages of practice, often the essence of the sacred object retreats, leaving only the mundane aspect in its place. This further encourages an already active mind to dwell in the ordinary, rather than set the sights on diving deep to the extraordinary.

As we become accustomed to traveling to these refined states of awareness, we must have both the insight and courage to move to the next stage in our quest. It is in this crucial time when even the most sacred meditation technique needs to be abandoned. These practices served as vehicles allowing us to traverse the seemingly endless bridge between individual and Divine Consciousness. Once we enter these exalted states, nothing can be brought with us. For many devoted students of meditation this is a difficult task. We become attached to our prayers, mantras, scriptures, etc. But it is necessary to let go of it all to venture to the wordless, objectless state of *Samadhi*.

My teacher, Sri Swami Satchidanandaji, often told a story about a fox that was infested with fleas. As it was impossible to get them out of its thick fur, a creative solution was required. Making its way to the river, the fox picked up a long stick and held it in its mouth. With slow, deliberate steps the fox waded into the river.

The pests, seeking refuge from the rising water level, climbed higher and higher in a feeble attempt to escape. Realizing their peril, they scampered upward, congregating first on the shoulders, then the neck, and finally the jaw. Feeling victory close at hand, the fox squatted, completely immersing its body in the river with only the stick remaining in the air. The fleas crawled onto the stick, thinking it a safe haven. The moment the fox could no longer feel the creatures in its fur, the stick where they now congregated was unceremoniously plunged into the water. Relieved of the discomfort and the fleas themselves, the fox left the moving water for the safety of the shore, feeling liberated.

And so it happens when we are at the threshold of higher consciousness: We leave everything good, bad, or neutral behind.

*Through the three phases of* **Samyama,** *the natural elements are transformed, as are the thoughts, feelings, and senses, securing and expanding the state of higher consciousness.*

CHAPTER

3

# THE MANIFESTATION OF POWER

I N THIS CHAPTER the *siddhis* or powers are expounded upon. It quickly becomes apparent that these *siddhis* are beyond the scope of the cognitive mind. The practices offered are not intended to invoke the *siddhis* but rather to cultivate an understanding and expand awareness of unlimited possibilities.

*An object possessing the external attributes of nature (gunas) remains subject to constant change, revealing the past, present, or yet to be manifested.*

*The progression of these attributes of nature is the cause of constant changes in our ongoing evolution.*

*From* Samyama *on the advancing of time comes knowledge of past and future.*

*A word, its meaning, and the idea behind it are often confused because of their superimposition upon one another. By* Samyama *on the word or sound, knowledge of its meaning is revealed.*

*Through* Samyama *on past impressions, knowledge of previous births is granted.*

*Through purity of consciousness, one gains the ability to understand the nature of their own mind and also those of others.*

*Understanding the nature of another's thoughts and feelings gives us insight into the contents and motives beyond them.*

*By* Samyama *on the subtle body, one gains the power to intercept the light emanating from their body before it reaches the eyes of the observer; therefore the yogi's body becomes invisible.*

*In the same way as described above, one is able to intercept the outward manifestation of the senses of smell, taste, hearing, and touch, so they become undetectable to others.*

*By* Samyama *on two aspects of karma (instantaneous and delayed), knowledge of the fruits of our actions will be revealed, along with time of death.*

*By* Samyama *on kindness and other virtuous qualities, one develops the power to transmit those qualities to others.*

*By* Samyama *on strength, we experience the level of vigor of elephants.*

*By* Samyama *on the inner light in the heart, one is granted powers of deep perception.*

III.14 *An object possessing the external attributes of nature* (gunas) *remains subject to constant change, revealing the past, present, or yet to be manifested.*

III.15 *The progression of these attributes of nature is the cause of constant changes in our ongoing evolution.*

III.16 *From* Samyama *on the advancing of time comes knowledge of past and future.*

Here again we meet the concept of the *trigunas,* the three attributes of nature: *Sattwa,* balance; *Rajas,* activity; and *Tamas,* inactivity (see page 14). Remember that the *gunas,* while present in all of nature, are found in varying proportions within each object, including our bodies and minds. These sutras describe the effects of the constantly changing *gunas* through the concept of time.

Because of the continual progression of the three *gunas,* all objects are influenced, keeping them in constant flux. Depending on how the *gunas* manifest, they may have an effect on furthering or hindering our ongoing evolution toward harmony and oneness.

Through *Samyama* on the advancing of time, we are able to balance the *gunas* and to understand how the past will impact the future.

*An object possessing the external attributes of nature* (gunas) *remains subject to constant change, revealing the past, present, or yet to be manifested.*

*The progression of these attributes of nature is the cause of constant changes in our ongoing evolution.*

*From* Samyama *on the advancing of time comes knowledge of past and future.*

## EXPERIENCING THE PAST AND FUTURE

*Assume a comfortable and relaxed sitting position.*

*Take in a few deep breaths and let them out slowly.*

*Begin to recall an event that took place in the past.*

*Bring forth all the details of the event, including who you were with, what you were wearing, and the topic of conversation.*

*Now bring forth in your mind an event that is similar in character that will happen in the future.*

*It could be a date with a friend, a business meeting, a holiday, anything that could repeat some of the same patterns as the event in the past.*

*Divide your mental screen and observe the past event on one side and the future event on the other.*

*Notice that you as the witness are in the middle between the two, resting in the present moment.*

*Make a mental note of any of the actions you would like to advance forward and the ones you would like to leave in the past.*

*When the* gunas *are in balance, we can both observe and influence the past and the future.*

III.17 *A word, its meaning, and the idea behind it are often confused because of their superimposition upon one another. By Samyama on the word or sound, knowledge of its meaning is revealed.*

This becomes a very important aspect in the worldly as well as the spiritual sense. It grants us the ability to intuit and understand what a person means rather than taking their words at face value. Many people have difficulty expressing their feelings and ideas simply using words. We even use the expression "I cannot find the words to express how I feel about this." This looms true especially when dealing with expressing heartfelt issues.

Some would categorize this *siddhi* as *mind reading,* a rare phenomenon. It is actually more commonplace than we imagine. Even at the outset of meeting, we may notice someone's slumped posture and assume they are a bit sad. Or their face may hold a certain expression trying to block an emotion from emerging. Yet when we greet them with "How are you?" they respond with "Oh, I am just fine."

They want you to think they are indeed fine, but the energy they are expressing does not back up that claim. If a smile and an open posture were present, their assertion might seem more legitimate.

I would often experience this when working with people with life-threatening diseases. When I would ask the obvious "How do you feel today?" the automatic response was often "Good." But careful observation advised me differently. When I gently prompted, "Are you *really* feeling good?" the truth often followed. With tear-filled eyes, they would ask, "Why is it that everyone else takes my words at face value, but *you* seem to go to the core? I am in pain and trying to hide it, but I guess not from you!" Is it a great *siddhi* or a honed observation arising from the heart that allows us to traverse the depth of another's soul? Or one and the same?

Reaching the state of *Samyama*, discernment dawns and the true meaning of word and sound is uncovered.

*A word, its meaning, and the idea behind it are often confused because of their superimposition upon one another. By* **Samyama** *on the word or sound, knowledge of its meaning is revealed.*

## EXPERIENCING THE TRUE MEANING BEHIND THE WORD OR SOUND

*Next time you are speaking with an acquaintance or friend, notice, without judgment, if their words match the vibration they are expressing.*

*When they say, "I am happy," do they look happy?*

*Does their physical posture express happiness? Does their voice reinforce that quality?*

*At first it may seem difficult to match what they are saying with the outward manifestation.*

*If appropriate, gently begin to ask them what is behind the way they hold their body or the expression on their face.*

*Sometimes there is great resistance on their part to share. Try opening your heart a bit more, and gently cajole them to speak about how they feel.*

*The more you refine your skills of observation, the more proficient you become at understanding the meaning within the word or sound.*

III.18 *Through* Samyama *on past impressions, knowledge of previous births is granted.*

III.19 *Through purity of consciousness, one gains the ability to understand the nature of their own mind and also those of others.*

III.20 *Understanding the nature of another's thoughts and feelings gives us insight into the contents and motives beyond them.*

Every experience we have starts from a ripple in the *chitta*. As the gross impressions subside, they become finer and finer but still remain in subtle form. When impressions resurface, it is termed memory. By *Samyama* on these past impressions, all past lives are remembered.

We are now introduced to the power of *clairvoyance,* the ability to see that which cannot be seen by the normal means of vision. We venture beyond our customary understanding to the inner workings of the mind, to the place where the hidden is revealed. The ability to see that which is concealed by the normal vision, *clairvoyance* can also be discovered as intuition.

Intuition does not belong to *clairvoyance* alone; it encompasses a number of the *siddhis*, including *clairaudience, clairsentience,* etc. Intuition is the quality expressed when the heart expands. This reaches beyond the boundaries of ordinary sensory output so we may discover the true essence of people, objects, and life.

The ability to read and understand minds is something many of us place in a carnival setting or on a TV show. Usually, the person doing the reading formulates a trick to determine the answers. It is the rare individual who possesses the ability to know the mind of another, a true *siddha*.

Some individuals have acquired this *siddhi* from a former incarnation. Often young children, with their uncluttered senses, are able to look into our souls and find answers and motives. As adults, we often doubt our innate psychic abilities, causing any remnant of them to recede. With the constant presence of spiritual practice these *siddhis* are refreshed and replenished.

We can easily understand how mother's intuition melds right in with these sutras. When we bond with and nurture a child, a form of *clairvoyance* is bestowed. Much to the child's chagrin, their mother seems to know what they are up to even from miles away. It is when intuition manifests through the sense of seeing that it is known as *clairvoyance*.

As with all aspects we wish to nourish, using it in everyday life brings it up close and personal.

*Through* **Samyama** *on past impressions, knowledge of previous births is granted.*

*Through purity of consciousness, one gains the ability to understand the nature of their own mind and also those of others.*

*Understanding the nature of another's thoughts and feelings gives us insight into the contents and motives beyond them.*

## EXPERIENCING CLAIRVOYANCE

*Try this practice multiple times with different people, and notice if you are able to interpret the motives beyond their thoughts, words, and feelings.*

*Sit with a friend and begin to "see" how their face and body looks when engaged in neutral conversation. Can you "see" what they are trying to express?*

*After a time, begin to bring up a more delicate, perhaps even an uncomfortable, topic.*

*Notice if their face and body shift when the subject changes from one of comfort to one of a more challenging nature.*

*Allow yourself to enter an experiential rather than thinking state.*

*Bypass your own opinions, focusing instead on how their spoken words and gestures evoke feelings within you.*

*It may bring about a subtle vibration in your body, or a visual image may appear.*

*Since you are beginning to develop your skills, file any observations in a corner of your mind rather than speaking them aloud.*

*In time,* clairvoyance *will become stronger and clearer and the truth will succeed.*

III.21 *By* Samyama *on the subtle body, one gains the power to intercept the light emanating from their body before it reaches the eyes of the observer; therefore the yogi's body becomes invisible.*

III.22 *In the same way as described above, one is able to intercept the outward manifestation of the senses of smell, taste, hearing, and touch, so they become undetectable to others.*

Imagine having the ability to be in a room where a conversation takes place and not be seen. This has interesting implications.

   Some years back I was coteaching with a spiritual teacher who was plagued with shyness when not in front of a class. When he entered the classroom, it was as if he was invisible until he reached the stage. In this way I was able to continue speaking without interruption. I exhibited the opposite quality, in that I would be *felt* by the students as soon as I entered the building. In that way they were able to anticipate my arrival in the classroom in advance of my physical entrance. We would often joke that he had the *siddhi* of being invisible, while my power allowed me to be present even when not physically there. Two *siddhis*, different intentions; both aspects can be useful.

*By* Samyama *on the subtle body, one gains the power to intercept the light emanating from their body before it reaches the eyes of the observer; therefore the yogi's body becomes invisible.*

*In the same way as described above, one is able to intercept the outward manifestation of the senses of smell, taste, hearing, and touch, so they become undetectable to others.*

III.23 *By* Samyama *on two aspects of karma (instantaneous and delayed), knowledge of the fruits of our actions will be revealed, along with time of death.*

Through common usage karma, known as cause and effect, has become synonymous with reward and punishment. Many believe that there is an egalitarian figure doling out good or bad karma to fit our every action. Even those of us who strive to *be good* will falter at some time or another. It is at those times we envision this benevolent judge, busy with someone else's transgressions, granting us a one-time pardon.

Karma, meaning action, can also be a reaction to an action. The response is not always equal *or* opposite in its intensity, as the original action is sometimes stronger, sometimes less. The reaction varies according to the intensity and vigilance of our spiritual practice. For that reason it is sometimes difficult to assess the ways of karma.

While at their origin most traditional religions adhere to the teachings of karma, it is often hidden from the believers for fear of misinterpretation. Some of these teachings, while clandestine, are difficult to ignore. There is a parable in the New Testament where the wise one is questioned as to why a baby was born blind. The onlooker asks, "Whose fault is it that the baby is blind? Is it the baby's or the father's fault?"

Interesting question from a religion that claims not to believe in reincarnation. If it was not the result of deeds in a previous birth, how is it possible for either the child *or* the parent to be responsible for the affliction? Although many may dismiss the teaching as irrelevant, its reference to karma and reincarnation cannot be denied.

Why do people question the validity of karma? Does knowing the laws of karma diminish the pain of a child being born sightless? For the astute follower, understanding the underlying cause can ease the suffering, as karma often provides context to many unexplained situations.

Attributing any blessing or tragedy to the law of karma does not absolve the perpetrator for their part in the incident. Nor is it a basis for excusing wrongdoing. Yet when understood as cause and effect, it has the ability to shed light on issues that seem impossible to comprehend. Throughout our lives every thought, feeling, and action will have input into determining which karma will come to fruition.

By *Samyama* on *ways of* karma, knowledge of the time of death is gained. With this advance knowledge the yogi has time to alter any actions that would determine the inevitability of rebirth. Therefore, knowing the time of death becomes essential.

*By* **Samyama** *on two aspects of karma (instantaneous and delayed), knowledge of the fruits of our actions will be revealed, along with time of death.*

---

### EXPERIENCING THE WORKINGS OF KARMA

*Sit quietly, and take in a few deep breaths.*

*Invite an important decision you are about to make into your awareness.*

*With the usual scrutiny you would give the topic, follow it through from its inception to its conclusion.*

*In your mind's eye, project how the various outcomes would affect your living situation, your relationships, your career, and ultimately your life, not only for the present but for years to come.*

*Along with the outer changes, how will your decision influence the flow of energy nourishing your spiritual path?*

*Be still and contemplate how the many different scenarios could play out. Is there one in particular that would create a positive effect?*

*After you have mapped out your strategy for moving ahead, open your eyes and take a moment to write it down.*

*Refer to your notes as you begin to reap the fruits of your actions.*

## III.24 *By* Samyama *on kindness and other virtuous qualities, one develops the power to transmit those qualities to others.*

When the ideal of kindness was first introduced (sutra 1.33, page 85), the concept offered an evolutionary practice toward oneness. On first glance the quality of kindness may not seem like a high spiritual virtue. Yet as we evaluate our encounters and relationships, this quality is often retracted or hidden. To be fully present with an open heart to another, in this age of quick encounters, is not only a virtue but a true gift. Book III transforms this precious concept from an aspiring practice into a state of being that has the power to transmit these exalted qualities to others.

When we allow our spiritual nature to direct our lives, kindness and compassion are elevated. It is important when choosing a focus for meditation that it elevates your mental and emotional states as well as reflects who you want to become. Choosing kindness and compassion allows us to express these qualities and invites them to be shared with many. In that way peace rests in our hearts.

A person burgeoning with kindness is welcomed everywhere. There is an immediate transformational quality they radiate to every person and situation they encounter.

The New York subway is not necessarily the place we think of to develop kindness, or *any* virtuous quality for that matter, yet for one evening rider, it did just that. It was the same train route that Inga always took at the end of a long workday. She was eager to arrive home, take off her shoes, put up her feet, and relax. Her body could almost feel the anticipated relaxation when a very curious little girl nestled up to her, needing some distraction from what appeared to be for her an arduous journey.

Inga responded with kindness, "Are you ready to go home, put on your pajamas, and go to bed?"

It might have been a projection on Inga's part, but it started a dialogue.

"What are pajamas?"

A bit startled by the response, Inga replied, "Pajamas are what you sleep in." A curious look appeared on the small face. "Don't you know what pajamas are? What do you sleep in?"

"I sleep in the underwear that I wore that day."

The statement prompted Inga to look more closely at the child. The tattered clothes revealed the reason pajamas were unknown. The girl's clothes had rips and tears and ground-in smudges from top to toe. Looking toward the mother, Inga detected a sense of embarrassment at the condition of her child's appearance.

A bit hesitant, Inga compassionately asked if she could send a gift of pajamas to the young girl from the store where she was employed. With some reluctance the mother wrote down the address where they would receive the gift.

The next day, while she was preparing to send the package, an idea occurred to Inga. If there was one child in need, there most likely were more. Her mission had begun. First she approached her employer for donations of children's sleepwear. Carrying the bundles to her apartment, she made a mental note of other nearby stores she could solicit. The stops proved fruitful, and soon her home was filled with bags of small-sized pj's.

She began to recruit her friends and neighbors to distribute the nightclothes to homeless shelters, schools, daycare centers, anywhere there was need. Inga was pleased with the enthusiasm of the recruits as they gladly distributed the clothing to delighted recipients. The local merchants learned of her efforts, and before long a warehouse was needed for all the donated items, which now included clothing for daytime, outerwear, and shoes. The hearts of the volunteers held images of the beaming faces of the children who dressed each night in their new "clothes," ready for bed.

One person's kindness to a small child evoked a deep compassion that inspired others to give. It is difficult to know who benefited more, the children in their new wardrobe or those who understood the joy of kindness through newfound compassion.

*By Samyama on kindness and other virtuous qualities, one develops the power to transmit those qualities to others.*

## EXPERIENCING KINDNESS

*Begin to bring the awareness to a time when you bestowed kindness on a particular person or situation.*

*Recall the person's face as they received your gift.*

*Do you remember the smile, the joy in their heart?*

*Begin to reflect how even this small kindness could have transformed their day or even their life.*

*Notice how good that feels in your body and heart.*

*Now bring back a time when you did not use this virtue and regretted it afterward.*

*Remember how the person looked and how it felt to you.*

*Could a different outcome have manifested if kindness had been applied?*

*If you cannot go back to remedy that situation in person, use your inner vision to visit the person with your open heart.*

*Express how you feel about them and offer the kindness missing the last time.*

*Notice how you feel.*

*Write down your thoughts and feelings; it will act as a reminder the next time life calls for these qualities.*

## III.25 *By* Samyama *on strength, we experience the level of vigor of elephants.*

The mere mention of these gentle giants brings to mind many of their qualities. Elephants are revered in many parts of the world, not only for their strength but also for their fortitude, their ability to relate to humans, and their wonderful memory.

We have all seen photos of these mighty beasts pulling huge loads with seemingly little effort. They have helped with the building of great halls and temples. Yet with all the power they possess, they can be very gentle and loving. But if they are provoked, stay clear and far from harm's way.

I recall visiting one of the great temples of India, where my guru, Sri Swami Satchidanandaji, served for many years as the temple manager. Each day as he entered the temple to perform his duties, the magnificent pachyderm in residence gently and lovingly blessed him by caressing the top of his head with her trunk. While her mighty trunk could have easily crushed him, elephants have the inherent ability to know just how much strength and power is needed in each situation. Even many years after he left his position at the temple, whenever Sri Swamiji returned, the great and mighty elephant remembered him with that same sweet, gentle caress.

Elephants have long been valued for their great strength and stamina while serving as the symbol of memory and power.

Recognizing the innate qualities of strength and resilience, many asanas were developed to cultivate these qualities. Noteworthy on this list is *tadasana,* mountain pose. This simple yet profound asana directs the energy downward through the feet and into the earth. This affords us a feeling of steadiness and strength. Grounding is something we can all benefit from in this fast-paced world we inhabit.

By Samyama *on strength, we experience the level of vigor of elephants.*

---

### EXPERIENCING MOUNTAIN POSE (*TADASANA*)

*Stand or sit in a chair with your feet firmly planted on the ground or floor.*

*Allow the arms to dangle by your sides.*

*Take a deep inhalation emanating from the belly, and with the exhalation send the breath downward through the body, through the legs, and out through the soles of the feet into the earth.*

*Repeat several times.*

*Hold steady in the pose for a few minutes.*

*By planting roots deep in the earth, the spirit is free to propel upward to the heavens.*

## III.26 *By* Samyama *on the inner light in the heart, one is granted powers of deep perception.*

As the power of perception is gained, it brings occult (hidden) objects and concepts once thought to be out of reach into view. With this renewed understanding of life and nature, perception expands exponentially, enabling us to comprehend the gross as well as the occult.

The wisdom of the Upanishads explains that there is a small flame that resides in each heart, the light of the True Self. When our heart's radiance becomes the beacon we follow, our relationships have the ability to traverse from casual to profound levels. Along with the Upanishads, most of the great religious traditions honor and expound upon the many virtues of living from the heart.

Do you know the expression "They have a dark heart"? This occurs when the heart becomes tainted, hindering the light from reflecting outward. The light in the heart becomes obscured when we are confused or plagued by disturbing thoughts or actions. If we hope to gain the power to delve into another's heart or intentions, our own heart must reflect purity, portraying a deep sense of trust.

This purity necessitates that the *Yamas* and *Niyamas,* the first two facets of *Asthaanga Yoga,* be respected and actualized. Adhering to the first *Yama, Ahimsa* (reverence for all), overrides any danger of acquiring this *siddhi* for selfish reasons or to do harm. It recognizes all hearts as *one* and perceives the same light in all.

**By** Samyama **on the inner light in the heart, one is granted powers of deep perception.**

# CONTINUING THE EXPLORATION OF *SAMYAMA*

HERE WE CONTINUE to explore as *Samyama* evokes the *siddhis* that are gifts along the way. These sutras hold the key to greater understanding, while the practical applications offered aid our ability to bring the powers partially or fully into a conscious life.

*By Samyama on the sun, knowledge of the inner and outer worlds is revealed.*

*By Samyama on the moon, we gain knowledge of the stars and galaxies as well as the subtle aspects of our being.*

*By Samyama on the polestar* (Dhruva Nakshatra) *comes knowledge of the celestial movements and their effects on the events of this world.*

*By Samyama on the navel, one acquires knowledge of how the human body functions and its constitution.*

*By Samyama at the base of the throat, the cessation of hunger and thirst is achieved.*

*By Samyama at the base of the throat, steadiness in meditation for both body and mind is accomplished.*

By Samyama *on the light radiating from the center of the head, visions of celestial and enlightened beings are bestowed.*

*Or all these powers and the knowledge within them may be imparted to those who become spontaneously enlightened through a life of purity.*

By Samyama *on the spiritual heart* (Hridaya), *the intent and contents of the* chitta *are revealed.*

*Through* Samyama *we are able to distinguish between the* chitta *and the True Self.*

*From this knowledge arise all our supernatural senses, which correspond to the external senses of sight, hearing, touch, taste, and smell.*

*While considered to be great accomplishments, these occult senses can be obstacles to reaching* Samadhi *and higher consciousness.*

III.27 *By* Samyama *on the sun, knowledge of the inner and outer worlds is revealed.*

We marvel at the celestial beauty of the sun, moon, planets, and stars expanding into the vastness of the cosmos. Yet most of us are unaware that there are celestial bodies encased within our being. By *Samyama* on the celestial sun, its potential power to uncover the mysteries is unveiled. From this realization the energy vortexes encased within our subtle bodies are empowered. It seems the further we venture outward into space, the more we are able to dive deep within.

The seven mystical energy vortexes, or chakras, through *Samyama* are revealed as portals of light that escort us beyond our worldly knowledge to the infinite universe.

The seven chakras manifest as whirling vortexes of energy and light. Intellectual knowledge alone is insufficient to understand or experience the chakras. When the subtle senses are refined and some level of spiritual evolution is present, these seven mystical vortexes become apparent. They can be *seen* by acquiring the *siddhi* of *clairvoyance, heard* with *clairaudience,* and *felt* with *clairsentience*.

The *Sahasara* chakra, at the crown of the head, facilitates a constant connection to our Divine Essence. At this, the highest level of awareness, the longing to reunite with our spiritual nature is continually present.

The energy emanating from the *Sahasara* forms the other six chakras. In descending order, the next three chakras—*Ajna* (brow point), *Vishudda* (throat), and *Anahatha* (heart)—manifest and are constant reminders that we are forever one with the cosmic energy.

*Manipura* (solar plexus), *Swadhisthana* (sacral plexus), and *Muladhara* (base) secure us to the earth. When the chakras are in balance, harmony governs every aspect of life. Each chakra can be understood as a self-effulgent aspect of the Divine Self. Or to explain it another way, each chakra is like the celestial sun.

*By Samyama on the sun, knowledge of the inner and outer worlds is revealed.*

## III.28 *By Samyama on the moon, we gain knowledge of the stars and galaxies as well as the subtle aspects of our being.*

This *siddhi* grants access to explore the night sky, peppered with planets, stars, and the far-reaching galaxies beyond.

The moon's energy greatly influences every aspect of our lives. Although thousands of miles away from Earth, the moon's movements and phases directly affect our mental and emotional states. Most of us have witnessed the effect the moon has on our moods and decisions, depending on whether it is full, new, waxing, or waning. It is well known that when it is at its zenith, the emotions peak, tempers flare, feelings are hurt. Also, as emergency room staff can attest, at the full moon accidents of all kinds become more prevalent.

This is understandable as we remember it is the moon's gravitational pull that moves mighty seas to slosh to and fro, producing the tides. If this energetic pull is so profound on the mighty oceans, how does it affect our bodies, composed of over 60 percent water? It is not a great leap to envision the same attraction that causes the tides to ebb and flow also impacting our mental and emotional states.

A woman's body is very much influenced by the moon. Her

reproductive phases mimic the moon's as it orbits through its twenty-eight-day cycle. Even the word "menses," as in "menstruation," comes from the same root word as "moon." The moon's energy induces the female of the species to produce a ripened egg once a month. And if the right time and circumstances are in play, when the egg and the sperm meet, a new life is created.

*By Samyama on the moon, we gain knowledge of the stars and galaxies as well as the subtle aspects of our being.*

## EXPERIENCING THE EFFECT OF THE CYCLES OF THE MOON ON YOUR MOOD

*Next time there is a full moon, try this practice.*

*For each of the three evenings prior to and including the full-moon night, find a place outside (or near a window) where you are fully bathed by Luna's light. Relax there for fifteen to twenty minutes.*

*The eyes may be closed or open, gazing at the moon.*

*Observe the movements of the mind.*

*Write down any significant thoughts or feelings that surface through all three nights.*

*Look at your entries and notice any similarities or differences among them.*

*With the onset of the new moon, initiate the practice as you did for the full moon. (Since the moon is not visible, allow yourself to be drawn into its darkness.)*

*For three days observe the movements of your mind each time you sit and observe. Note them.*

*At the end of both periods, compare your journal writing.*

*Are there any similarities between the two periods as a whole? Is one more active than the other?*

*If you are really keen, try doing this not only on the full or new moon but for a full month to evaluate how the moon affects your mood.*

*You might find that you have garnered a new respect for the moon's cycles.*

**III.29** *By* Samyama *on the polestar (*Dhruva Nakshatra*) comes knowledge of the celestial movements and their effects on the events of this world.*

This wonderful sutra encourages us to look to the stars for universal knowledge. The systems of astrology, both Eastern (Jyotish/Indian) and Western, give us insights into how the celestial movements affect us individually and as a society. *Samyama* on the polestar reveals the planets' hold on our destiny and the inner secrets of the cosmos.

The planets are continually transmitting their wisdom; it is up to us to learn their language. Performing *Samyama* on the polestar grants us an understandable and translatable insight into the mysteries of the celestial bodies and their effect on us.

On my first visit to an Ayurvedic clinic in India, in order to begin treatment, the astrology charts had to be formulated. The physicians and therapists awaited the results of the reading to determine which cures were needed and when to begin. When this protocol was adhered to, the medical team was assured that the efficacy of the treatments would be enhanced.

*By Samyama on the polestar (Dhruva Nakshatra) comes knowledge of the celestial movements and their effects on the events of this world.*

### III.30 *By Samyama on the navel, one acquires knowledge of how the human body functions and its constitution.*

This sutra references the navel, which as a physical attribute does not hold mystical powers. It might be clearer to identify it in its subtle form as the *Manipura* chakra, located *at the solar plexus,* rather than by its location and attributes. When sourced, this chakra reveals the intricacies of the human body and how to rebalance it when it becomes unstable.

The *Manipura* chakra manifests as a resplendent source of power, reminiscent of the sun at the center of the celestial system. This power affords the ability to understand the functioning of the body and discloses how we think, reason, experience, learn, and enjoy great vitality.

*By Samyama on the navel, one acquires knowledge of how the human body functions and its constitution.*

## EXPERIENCING THE *MANIPURA* CHAKRA AT THE SOLAR PLEXUS

*Allow the body and mind to become quiet, the eyes to close.*

*Begin to venture to the* Manipura *chakra, the energy center located at the solar plexus.*

*There, awaiting your awareness, is a glowing energy reminiscent of the sun.*

*Observe that energy as it awakens the understanding of how the body and its constitution function.*

*Using this keen perception, begin to observe the energy as it flows through*
*the arms . . .*
*through the torso to the vital organs . . .*
*through the head and organs of senses . . .*
*down through the legs to the feet.*

*In this way we become acquainted with the gross aspects of the human body.*

*Leaving the physical aspect, notice how the subtle energy empowers the body to function efficiently and powerfully.*

*As we move to the mind, the same energy now enhances the power of intellect.*

*Recognize the* Manipura *chakra as a transmitter of energy powered by the internal sun.*

*The more powerful the energy, the easier it is to think and understand new concepts.*

*It is honored when we honor our own power.*

### III.31 *By* Samyama *at the base of the throat, the cessation of hunger and thirst is achieved.*

### III.32 *By* Samyama *at the base of the throat, steadiness in meditation for both body and mind is accomplished.*

At the base of the throat, we find the *Vishudda* (purity) chakra. It manifests the rarefied ether element that has the ability to propel us beyond the earth's jurisdiction. Ether, being the most refined of the earth's elements, is known in its subtlest form as *prana*. *Prana* is the elusive, ever-present universal life force that asks us to take a leap of faith through understanding. It permeates and inhabits the natural world while infusing every cell of the physical body with this universal energy.

On the subtle level, also located at the base of the throat we find the *Kurma Nadi*. This *Nadi* (astral tube) carries *prana* and engages directly with the *Vishudda Chakra*. This *Nadi* is activated during *pranayama* and enhanced by *Jalandhara Bhanda*, the chin lock.

Hunger and thirst, being essential to our physical survival, often take precedence over our spiritual quest. Cravings for food and drink, when fueled by desires, satisfy the palate rather than simply nurturing the body. Here we are cautioned that if we do not use discrimination to limit our intake of essential food and drink, we remain at the mercy of our desires.

Through deep meditation we are freed from the cravings of hunger and thirst, allowing the energy that would be diverted to digestion, absorption, and elimination to be channeled into spiritual pursuits. In this way the mind, unable to fixate on gross movements, simultaneously diverts all energy of the body and mind inward, creating total stillness.

*By Samyama at the base of the throat, the cessation of hunger and thirst is achieved.*

*By Samyama at the base of the throat, steadiness in meditation for both body and mind is accomplished.*

## III.33 *By Samyama on the light radiating from the center of the head, visions of celestial and enlightened beings are bestowed.*

The focus of *Samyama* has now shifted to the energy vortex in the center of the head, the *Ajna* chakra, the eye of wisdom. This chakra manifests the universal truth of unity, outshining the duality that impacts our everyday consciousness. At its core it reveals the basic knowledge that *we are one* with everything,

Through the *Ajna* chakra we are blessed with many visions. The masters, saints, and enlightened beings are able to reach us with their light and wisdom when this chakra is illuminated. They impart wisdom gained from deep stages of *Samadhi* and, when summoned through the *Ajna* chakra, reveal it to us.

Often they will simply say, "Sit and be still. The wisdom will be revealed to you."

*By Samyama on the light radiating from the center of the head, visions of celestial and enlightened beings are bestowed.*

## EXPERIENCING MEDITATION
## ON THE *AJNA* CHAKRA

*Begin by placing a photo or statue of a great master, saint, or enlightened being of any tradition (or any image that emanates a spiritual essence) in front of you at eye level.*

*Bring the awareness to the third eye in the center of the forehead emanating as the Ajna chakra.*

*Slowly open the eyes halfway, allowing them to remain relaxed and soft.*

*Begin to gaze at the divine representation.*

*When ready, gently close the eyes.*

*Observe the image as seen by the inner vision.*

*As the image begins to fade, allow the eyes to open and gaze outward once again.*

*After a few minutes, allow the eyes to close, drawing deep within.*

*Be still as the image floods your entire being, illuminated through the dawning of the inner light.*

*By connecting to the universal consciousness, we experience oneness with all.*

**III.34** *Or all these powers and the knowledge within them may be imparted to those who become spontaneously enlightened through a life of purity.*

We have all met people who have extraordinary insight, wisdom, or even *siddhis* yet have never had a formal spiritual practice. Here we are encouraged to live a virtuous and pure life. To live consciously with grace and love, we align with our righteous path, or dharma. The basic precepts of Yoga encourage us to embrace *Ahimsa*, love and compassion for all, along with the other *Yamas* and *Niyamas*. Their message seems so basic, yet when adhered to, they have the transformative power to purify and elevate.

*Or all these powers and the knowledge within them may be imparted to those who become spontaneously enlightened through a life of purity.*

**III.35** *By* Samyama *on the spiritual heart (*Hridaya*), the intent and contents of the* chitta *are revealed.*

This sutra explains that the most direct route to the mind comes through the heart. Yet many of the interpretations of the higher spiritual teachings tend to relegate that authority to the mind. Living through the heart is not always a comfortable path, as the heart is tender and easily affected by negativity. However, the rewards of heart-centered living are vast, as it benefits both the giver and the receiver.

I was invited to speak on Yoga therapy at a university that was hosting a group of medical professionals from India. It was not my usual audience, and the high scrutiny of what I was about to present instilled a sense of caution. I chose to speak on consciousness emanating from the heart and based the discourse on the second sutra of Patanjali's Yoga Sutras, "*Yogah Chitta Vritti Nirodaha.*" Researching many translations, I found that the common ones said the path to Yoga was through controlling the mind.

The Upanishads, which predate the Yoga Sutras, state that consciousness resides in the *heart*. From that moment, for me, the translation of sutra 1.2 became "Yoga is the uniting of consciousness in the heart." The heart then becomes the source to reveal the mind's contents.

The talk was going well until a few listeners started to contest my translation of the sutra, as it was based on the heart, not the mind. It seemed it was necessary for them to expand their hearts to fully understand the concept. I asked them to close their eyes and focus on their spiritual hearts. The room suddenly became charged with a palpable feeling of connection, caring, and love. Finishing with a prayer for world peace, I took my leave of the stage enveloped in the indescribable feeling of joy in the room.

Later that day, I was approached by an Indian guru dressed in white. "My name is Shastraji," he said. "I am sorry to have missed your talk." I was a bit humbled to be noticed by a great teacher. He continued, "I heard what you did with the group, how they were transformed by love. That is not easy to do with such an audience. Did you know you were a *Prem Siddha* [having the power to transmit divine love]?"

It was a gift I did not know I had until it sprang forth when the field was fertile. It left me wondering how many of us could have such powers, still dormant, ready to blossom with the right circumstances.

The next time I met Shastraji was in India. He asked me what I was doing now that the cardiac research I was involved in was ending. A bit reticent, I shyly told him I was writing a translation of the Yoga Sutras from a heart-centered, woman's perspective. With a big smile he said, "It is about time!" And so, with his blessings, *The Secret Power of Yoga* was written.

*By* Samyama *on the spiritual heart* (Hridaya), *the intent and contents of the* chitta *are revealed.*

## EXPERIENCING MEDITATION
## ON THE SPIRITUAL HEART (*HRIDAYA*)

*Close the eyes, and feel yourself softening into a deep stillness and peace.*

*Bring the awareness to the* Anahatha *chakra, our connection to the forces of intuition, love, and compassion.*

*Observe how when the heart beats, love flows outward, and as the heart rests, love flows back to the heart.*

*With each inhalation, observe the capacity to receive love in the heart expand.*

*On the exhalation, allow that love to flow outward to someone you know who may need that loving energy, or offer it as a gift to the world.*

*As you inhale, the love deepens and, on the exhale, surround them with this love.*

*If there is a message to accompany this loving energy, send it silently.*

*Slowly and gently begin to bring the awareness back to your own heart, the source for universal love and compassion.*

*As love flows from its eternal source, it amplifies greatly when shared.*

## III.36 *Through* Samyama *we are able to distinguish between the* chitta *and the* True Self.

The spiritual adept is able to distinguish between the *chitta* and the True Self at their essence, while to the novice the two appear to be the same. Deep discernment is necessary when our limited experience concludes that they *are* one. If *Avidya* (absence of knowledge) comes into play, it overrides the discrimination needed to distinguish between the *chitta* and the True Self. As we advance in our spiritual understanding, the powers of discrimination reveal the differences between the two.

The comparison can be equated to the relationship between the sun and the moon. Both appear to be illumined. But in fact, the moon is not self-effulgent; it only appears to be a source of light through the reflection of the sun. It is the sun, not the moon, that is the source of light.

By performing *Samyama* on the distinction between the *chitta* and the True Self, knowledge of our divine essence is gained. This knowledge revealed during *Samyama* confirms that the *chitta*, in perpetual fluctuation, forgets its origin, while the True Self is constantly aware of its divine nature.

**Through** Samyama *we are able to distinguish between the* chitta *and the True Self.*

III.37 *From this knowledge arise all our supernatural senses, which correspond to the external senses of sight, hearing, touch, taste, and smell.*

III.38 *While considered to be great accomplishments, these occult senses can be obstacles to reaching* Samadhi *and higher consciousness.*

Recognizing the difference between *chitta* and the True Self, we are freed from the hold of the senses. The ordinary senses enable us to live life with fullness and vitality. As they are essential to life in our everyday sensory world, if even one of the senses is diminished, we face challenges in accomplishing the simplest daily chores. A person who is sightless calls upon the other senses to allow them to "see." They may use a cane to *feel* or *hear* sounds assuring them it is safe to cross the street or alerting them of any danger.

With recognition of the True Self, the extraordinary senses (clairvoyance, clairaudience, clairsentience, etc.) are empowered and become as available as the ones in constant use.

With this acquisition we are able to see, hear, touch, taste, and smell that which is undetected by the ordinary and limited senses.

Intrigued by this extrasensory perception, we glimpse future happenings or inhale the scent of blooming roses in midwinter. Most believe these *siddhis* are granted to the very few yet are delighted when, after years of spiritual practice, they emerge. While these feats may seem extraordinary, they become an integrated part of the fabric of our life as we spiritually evolve.

Even as we appreciate all the services our gross and subtle senses render to us, they create desires that then become obstacles to enlightenment. Instead of our being under *their* spell, they can be reoriented to serve us in our spiritual quest.

*From this knowledge arise all our supernatural senses, which correspond to the external senses of sight, hearing, touch, taste, and smell.*

*While considered to be great accomplishments, these occult senses can be obstacles to reaching* Samadhi *and higher consciousness.*

# THE ELEMENTS

THIS CLUSTER OF sutras expounds upon the relationship between *Samyama* and the elements of nature (*gunas*). As we are inherently created from nature as well as the Divine, it is prudent to understand the relationship between the two.

*Through loosening the bonds of karma, one can leave their body at will or even enter another's body.*

*By* Samyama *on the element of air, levitation over all naturally occurring objects, including water and land, becomes possible. It also grants the ability to die at will.*

*By* Samyama *on the solar plexus, the element of fire, housed there, causes the* samana vayu *(the equalizing vital air) to produce a radiant aura that surrounds the body.*

*By* Samyama *on the relationship between space and sound, one acquires the power of hearing distant and divine sounds; supernormal hearing (clairaudience) becomes possible.*

*By* Samyama *on the relationship between the body and ether, weightlessness and levitation are attained and traveling through space becomes possible.*

By Samyama *on consciousness* (Mahavideha), *the* chitta *acts independently from the physical body, causing the veil over the inner light of the Self to become transparent.*

By Samyama *on the basic and subtle characteristics of the natural elements and the* gunas *that comprise them, their purpose is revealed, and one gains mastery over them.*

By gaining mastery over the natural elements, one is no longer subjected to their play or the obstacles they impose on the physical body, allowing the eight supernatural powers to manifest.

Achieving this mastery, the physical body reveals beauty and grace, combined with solidity and strength.

III.39 *Through loosening the bonds of karma, one can leave their body at will or even enter another's body.*

What is keeping us tethered to karma? We need to look no further than the *Kleshas* (II.3–11, page 128) as the cause of bondage to the human form. These great obstacles to enlightenment directly affect all thoughts and feelings, dictating the way we live. Unveiling the knowledge that has been restricted by *Avidya,* the primary *Klesha,* we begin to comprehend the intricacies of karma. With the loosening of these bonds, the accomplished yogi gains the ability to leave their body or inhabit another body at will.

In the same way, much of the knowledge gained in present and previous births adheres to the soul as it traverses through its evolutionary path into the next incarnation.

**Through loosening the bonds of karma, one can leave their body at will or even enter another's body.**

III.40 *By Samyama on the element of air, levitation over all naturally occurring objects, including water and land, becomes possible. It also grants the ability to die at will.*

This *siddhi* allows the body to become so light it defies gravity by levitating above an object without physical contact. This mastery is realized when *Samyama* focuses on the *udana vayu* (the upward movement of *prana*). Much of this power stems from a combination of the air element housed in the *Anahatha* (heart) chakra and the ether element in the *Vishudda* (throat) chakra. The credit is shared, as to break contact with the earth's gravity, we must become lighter than air. This *siddhi* for levitation will reappear as one of the eight *siddhis*: *becoming as light as a feather*.

As we gain power over the upward *prana*, the ability to permanently separate from the physical body becomes under our control. This is accomplished by directing the *prana* to ascend through the *brahmarandhra nadi*, the entrance to the Divine. While this *nadi* is located within the subtle body, its physical parallel would lie near the hollow at the crown of the head known as the fontanel, the soft spot on a newborn baby. With maturity the bones of the skull fuse, and the sacred spot is concealed. For the advanced yogi, the moment of death signals this portal to fling open. It welcomes the dynamic energy as it ascends through the *Shushumna nadi* (central channel), arriving at the entrance to the divine realm, where the spirit reunites with its essence.

A hundred and one are the nerves of the heart. Of them only the *Shushumna* rises piercing the head and continues beyond. With this one attains immortality.

—*Katha Upanishad*

By Samyama *on the element of air, levitation over all naturally occurring objects, including water and land, becomes possible. It also grants the ability to die at will.*

III.41 *By* Samyama *on the solar plexus, the element of fire, housed there, causes the* samana vayu *(the equalizing vital air) to produce a radiant aura that surrounds the body.*

*Samana vayu* originates at the solar plexus, where the *prana vayu* (inward/upward) and *apana vayu* (outward/downward) join. The *samana vayu* is the bridge between the two opposing energies.

Before being refined through *Samyama,* the *apana vayu* projects all aspects of *chitta* outward, including thoughts, feelings, and senses, whether they be negative or positive.

The *prana vayu* governs *Agni,* the inward fire, essential for digestion, normally relegated to the processing of food. Channeling the *Agni* toward spiritual pursuits it transforms into the more subtle *Ojas.* Continuing to refine, *Tejas* comes forth as a brilliant radiance surrounding the entire being, the aura.

When this conversion occurs, the purified aura radiates only spiritual qualities.

*By* Samyama *on the solar plexus, the element of fire, housed there, causes the* samana vayu *(the equalizing vital air) to produce a radiant aura that surrounds the body.*

### EXPERIENCING MEDITATION
### ON THE SACRED FLAME

*Sit in front of a live fire or, if one is not available, place a candle directly in front of you.*

*Close the eyes. Take in a few deep breaths.*

*Slowly open the eyes and gaze at the flame.*

*Feel the warmth and light of the flame enter through your eyes. Guide it as it moves downward to meet the sun within you, at the solar plexus.*

*Reaching the solar plexus, observe the fire as it expands and pulsates outward, creating a glowing aura.*

*Allow all thoughts of love, compassion, harmony, and balance to be routed through the solar plexus, satiating the aura completely.*

*Radiating outward, these qualities embrace all with love and compassion.*

*Make a silent affirmation to nurture this purified energy so it may bless and benefit all.*

III.42 *By* Samyama *on the relationship between space and sound, one acquires the power of hearing distant and divine sounds; supernormal hearing (clairaudience) becomes possible.*

Many of us are blessed with the ability to hear external sounds. The songs of birds, a baby cooing, and even our neighbor's music can be cause for gratitude. Yet very few of us are aware that this precious ability harbors an even greater gift. By *Samyama* on the relationship between space and sound, the *Vishudda* chakra's ability to transform ordinary hearing into clairaudience awakens.

Clairaudience is the ability to hear that which cannot be heard through the physical ears or ordinary hearing. It also grants us the power to understand concepts beyond the jurisdiction of the mind. We often "hear" a warning that others do not or know the phone will ring moments before the actual sound. These bewildering events can cause discomfort for those who choose to rationalize them away or allow them to quickly be forgotten. Yet these are as much a part of us as our ordinary physical hearing. The subtler aspects of the senses tend to be shier and more easily taunted by our doubts, causing them to retreat. If we are able to welcome these gifts and honor their uses, they will strengthen and become constant companions, opening us to worlds only imagined!

It is important to understand the relationship between sound and space. When a sound is created, it travels from its source though the ether to reach the sensory receptor of hearing, the outer ear. Reaching its interim goal, it swirls around the external ear, eventually finding its way into the canal and to its final destination, the brain. Here the vibration is identified as sound and, if the memory finds a recognizable match, labeled. A long journey for a bird's chirp.

Clairaudience bypasses the external receptors of normal hearing, transporting us to a place where sounds are not dependent on cause *or* effect. We then gain the power to tap into celestial warnings, others' conversations, or events yet to happen. This *siddhi* can prove very useful even in everyday life.

There are many accounts of people about to board an airplane who, when cautioned by an ethereal voice to "make other arrangements," heeded the warning and were rewarded by news of delays or worse. "Don't take the freeway," my friend was cautioned. "That is ridiculous. It is so much quicker," the rational mind retorted. When stalled for more than an hour in traffic, she wondered why she had not listened to the quiet message. The more we honor clairaudience, the easier it is to access at will.

Also within this sutra the power of mantra (sutras 1.27–28, page 76) is acknowledged. A mantra can be a whole or partial word or sound that conveys a particular spiritual vibration.

Through mantra repetition, we gain the ability to traverse the bridge leading from the conscious to the superconscious or even beyond to the True Self. The scriptures offer three main ways to practice *japa,* the repetition of a mantra. With both heart and mind affixed to the sound, begin to repeat it aloud for a time. When you feel it vibrating in every cell, repeat silently with lip movements. When well established, repeat the mantra in silence, engaging only the mind and heart. The sacred sound, when continuously repeated, merges with the singular vibration of the universe, known as *Pranava*.

At a certain stage it becomes unnecessary to *repeat* the mantra; rather we *listen* as the sound continues to repeat into infinity. Spontaneous repetition of the mantra without mental involvement is known as *ajapa*. *Ajapa* is considered an aspect of clairaudience.

*By* Samyama *on the relationship between space and sound, one acquires the power of hearing distant and divine sounds; supernormal hearing (clairaudience) becomes possible.*

## III.43 *By* Samyama *on the relationship between the body and ether, weightlessness and levitation are attained and traveling through space becomes possible.*

This is another example of uniting with the power of the ether element. Sutra III.40 (page 337) spoke of a similar principle. Here the sutras reiterate that by *Samyama* we are able to make our bodies weightless, and the ability to float up and even propel ourselves to another location, whether here on earth or in the vast universe, is possible. This seemingly inconceivable accomplishment is actualized through harnessing the power of the ether element.

*By* Samyama *on the relationship between the body and ether, weightlessness and levitation are attained and traveling through space becomes possible.*

III.44 *By* Samyama *on consciousness* (Mahavideha), *the* chitta *acts independently from the physical body, causing the veil over the inner light of the Self to become transparent.*

*Mahavideha* is an interesting concept meaning the disembodied state. Through *Samyama* consciousness becomes autonomous from the physical body and gains the ability to function independently. This separation prompts the *Rajas* and *Tamas guna* to dwindle away, revealing the light of the *Sattwa guna*.

*By* Samyama *on consciousness* (Mahavideha), *the* chitta *acts independently from the physical body, causing the veil over the inner light of the Self to become transparent.*

III.45 *By* Samyama *on the basic and subtle characteristics of the natural elements and the* gunas *that comprise them, their purpose is revealed, and one gains mastery over them.*

III.46 *By gaining mastery over the natural elements, one is no longer subjected to their play or the obstacles they impose on the physical body, allowing the eight supernatural powers to manifest.*

Gaining power over nature and the three *gunas* (*Sattwa, Rajas,* and *Tamas*), we gain unrestricted access to all levels of awareness, as the elements no longer hold sway.

This part is reflective of the passage in chapter 2 of the Bhagavad Gita, where we are clearly given the limitations of the body as opposed to the unlimited aspects of the soul.

Sri Krishna describes the immortality of the soul:—

*Fire does not burn it; water does not wet it and wind does not dry it. —II.23*

*The Self cannot be pierced or cut. It cannot be burned, wetted, or dried. It is endless, all pervading, stable, immovable, and everlasting. —II.24*

The eight major *siddhis* manifest when they are no longer restricted by the natural elements. Some of these attributes have been described in earlier sutras. Here they are presented as a complete package, allowing us to cultivate one or more at a time.

I have offered some examples of how even our world, constrained by nature, portrays these great powers. While these worldly accomplishments are not exact equivalents of the *siddhis,* they need not be discounted. They could be worldly stepping-stones to the great powers. For some, these great feats are due to accomplishments in an earlier incarnation.

## THE EIGHT MAJOR *SIDDHIS*

*ANIMA SIDDHI:* to become very small
This has been parodied in films and books. We may see images of people shrunk down to comfortably fit into a blood vessel exploring the body. But if alchemy is mismanaged, they may remain that size. While these depictions are made in jest, there is a *siddhi* that can do just that. In fact, one can become the size of an atom.

One outcome is produced via special effects, the other is a *siddhi* granted by longtime, deep spiritual practice.

*MAHIMA SIDDHI:* to become very big
Returning to fantasy, we have seen average-sized people burst their seams to become huge, towering over tall buildings. These special effects evoke a range of emotions that seem possible only if it were an actual event that we witnessed.

In the eleventh chapter of the Bhagavad Gita the cosmic form is revealed to a stunned Arjuna, who has known Sri Krishna only in human form. Knowing it is impossible to compress the Divine into human proportions, Sri Krishna invokes this *siddhi* enabling Arjuna to envision him in his cosmic form. Sri Krishna's modest human form spontaneously grows to such enormity that one eye becomes the sun while the other eye is the moon. It is only with this exaggerated image that we are able to begin to comprehend the vastness and infinite nature of the Divine.

*GARIMA SIDDHI:* to become very heavy
As one gains proficiency in this *siddhi,* the ability to make the body very heavy is gained. Certain martial arts tout this particular *siddhi* as way of showing proficiency in the practice.

A famous master of Tai Chi challenged his students to try pushing him over. As he assumed a firm stance, the challengers smiled, thinking it was not a contest for their advanced skills. At first, their efforts were gentle, as they did not want to harm the master. It soon became obvious that the master was rooted to the earth by some unseen force. Moving him was as arduous as pushing a hippopotamus onto its side.

*LAGHIMA SIDDHI:* to become very light
This *siddhi* is one that many dancers strive to master, yet very few have perfected it. Enraptured by a graceful lift in ballet, we often

wonder how a person of average height and build is able to propel a fully grown adult over their head while in constant motion. The skill required to do this takes much practice and concentration. Imagining they are light as a feather, the dancer creates a body that is lithe and limber, with the ability to float upward, defying gravity. With any distraction, even for a moment, the effect dissipates.

I was excited to be at a performance of *Swan Lake* featuring one of the greatest dancers of our time. The dance troupe touted a stellar reputation for excellence, especially for their captivating lightness and grace in movement. All at once from stage left, seemingly out of thin air, this magnificent being sailed upward, propelled through the air across the stage, ultimately landing with the grace of an eagle. A profound silence followed an audible gasp as the spellbound audience released the breath captured by the performance. It was clear at that moment that the maestro, after years of meditating on the choreography, was no longer dancing; he had *become the dance*.

*PRAPTI SIDDHI:* to instantaneously travel at will
This *siddhi* is like a fairy godmother; it grants the ability to go anywhere we desire. Nothing is too great or impossible for one who has gained this power. Imagine craving a flaky croissant and voilà, you are sitting at a café in Paris. A peaceful beach? Gather your swimwear, because instantly you are at the seaside. Be careful what you wish for; if you acquire this *siddhi,* you just might get it!

*PRAKAMYA SIDDHI:* to realize whatever one desires
This *siddhi* grants the ability to develop and become whatever we choose. The only limitation is our imagination. By directing the supernatural energies toward her priorities and desires, the *siddha* does or becomes anything she yearns for. Here the sky is *not* the limit!

*ISHITA SIDDHI:* to gain supremacy over nature and to influence anyone or anything

This takes the idea of persuasion to an extreme. Here we are given the ominous power to influence the behavior of individuals, groups, or even nations. We can understand why *Yama* and *Niyama* are always encouraged first and foremost. This could be a dangerous power in the hands of the unrefined practitioner. One accommodating perk with this *siddhi* is the ability to change the weather. Those holiday picnics and outdoor concerts would never be rained out! Expanding the scope of this *siddhi,* we gain control over *all* the elements.

*VASHITA SIDDHI:* to gain life-and-death control over all living things

This *siddhi* grants control over our bodies and minds, the environment, our work, friends, and family. The power allows us to control our own destiny and determine how and when we die. Once achieved, it demands great responsibility. With the help of this *siddhi,* we attain control over all living beings. The one who excels in this *siddhi* has great influence over any person or object on this earth.

**By** Samyama *on the basic and subtle characteristics of the natural elements and the* gunas *that comprise them, their purpose is revealed, and one gains mastery over them.*

*By gaining mastery over the natural elements, one is no longer subjected to their play or the obstacles they impose on the physical body, allowing the eight supernatural powers to manifest.*

III.47 *Achieving this mastery, the physical body reveals beauty and grace, combined with solidity and strength.*

Each year millions of dollars are doled out for one reason: to procure a body of perfect beauty, health, and strength. We spend money on wrinkle creams, expensive exercise equipment, natural and nutritious food, all with the same goal. We strive to create a body that defies the play of the natural elements; we even resort to surgical procedures to fool our friends and co-workers. The only one we cannot fool is nature itself.

When mastery of the *siddhis* that govern the natural elements is gained, the beauty and grace we dream of become a reality.

*Achieving this mastery, the physical body reveals beauty and grace, combined with solidity and strength.*

# CHAPTER 6

# *SAMYAMA* AND THE SENSES

IN THE LAST chapter we explored how *Samyama* interacts with and affects the elements of nature. We now study another aspect of *Samyama*, gaining mastery over the senses. Practices are offered to entice the senses to pivot inward.

> By Samyama *on the transformation that the senses undergo when they contact objects, and the experience they provide for the individual, mastery over the senses is gained.*

> *Thus the body gains the power to move as rapidly as thought, and the sense organs engage outside the confines of the body, enabling mastery over the aspects of nature* (Prakriti).

> *By recognizing the distinction between the* chitta *and the True Self, one gains knowledge of everything that exists and all that manifests within nature* (Prakriti).

> *After acquiring all these* siddhis, *if we renounce them, embracing only the Divine Self, liberation follows.*

III.48 *By* Samyama *on the transformation that the senses undergo when they contact objects, and the experience they provide for the individual, mastery over the senses is gained.*

The senses by nature are attracted to worldly objects and ways; this causes a yearning for constant interaction. If the senses are not appeased, the mind and emotions become agitated. If they are pacified, temporary calmness can be experienced. When the senses are aroused, if we resist the temptation to engage them, they begin to turn inward. This divergence is orchestrated by the higher intelligence trying to quell the outer enticements, in order to explore the inner realms. As a result, the senses and mind relinquish the duties of the outer world, resting permanently in the abode of the soul.

*By* Samyama *on the transformation that the senses undergo when they contact objects, and the experience they provide for the individual, mastery over the senses is gained.*

III.49 *Thus the body gains the power to move as rapidly as thought, and the sense organs engage outside the confines of the body, enabling mastery over the aspects of nature (*Prakriti*).*

By *Samyama* the ordinary senses are replaced in function with extrasensory perception, as previously described. We are now able to experience *clairvoyance* (seeing what the eyes cannot see), *clairaudience* (hearing what the ears cannot hear), and *clairsentience* (feeling energy).

*Thus the body gains the power to move as rapidly as thought, and the sense organs engage outside the confines of the body, enabling mastery over the aspects of nature* (Prakriti).

III.50 *By recognizing the distinction between the* chitta *and the True Self, one gains knowledge of everything that exists and all that manifests within nature* (Prakriti).

Here we become acquainted with the power of *omnipotence* and *omniscience*. Omnipotence is the quality of having unlimited power. Omniscience grants us infinite awareness, understanding, and insight. In these states we lose interest in external sensual gratification and pleasure, imbuing only the essence of the True Self.

*By recognizing the distinction between the* chitta *and the True Self, one gains knowledge of everything that exists and all that manifests within nature* (Prakriti).

III.51 *After acquiring all these* siddhis, *if we renounce them, embracing only the Divine Self, liberation follows.*

While it is tempting to delve into and conquer the psychic powers, we are again warned that they can lead us astray. They are summoned by our past experiences to fulfill any and all desires, similar to making a wish or daydreaming. Once these *siddhis* are realized, if they are then renounced as obstacles to enlightenment, liberation is granted.

*After acquiring all these* siddhis, *if we renounce them, embracing only the Divine Self, liberation follows.*

# EQUANIMITY

T HE REMAINING SUTRAS in *Vibhuti Pada* advise us that liberation is imminently on the horizon. Now we must choose a lifestyle that is in harmony with our newly elevated consciousness. The decision must be considered: whether to live in the world but not be a part of it, or to withdraw completely from society in order to continue to foster the bliss that is our birthright, or a combination of both. Whatever our choice, equanimity must be our guiding light.

*Dwelling in a state of equanimity, the yogi neither accepts nor rejects admiration from others, even celestial beings; thus their heart stays pure and embraces only the Divine.*

*By Samyama on the smallest moment, as well as the succession of moments of time, the knowledge of supreme liberation is attained.*

*With this exalted knowledge, the yogi is able to clearly distinguish even the most minute differences between two similar objects.*

*This intuitive knowledge, which has the ability
to comprehend all objects under various conditions
simultaneously, leads us to freedom.*

*Liberation is attained when the spiritual heart (Hridaya)
attains purity equal to that of the True Self.*

III.52 *Dwelling in a state of equanimity, the yogi neither accepts nor rejects admiration from others, even celestial beings; thus their heart stays pure and embraces only the Divine.*

Equanimity is a concept at the center of a yogi's existence. The Bhagavad Gita continually expresses the idea that *equanimity is Yoga*. Why is the concept of balance in one's life so essential to the spiritual seeker?

The path of Yoga, and indeed much of the quest for higher consciousness, has been likened to walking on the razor's edge. The razor-thin line tolerates only the most minute movement in either direction. Straying off center for even a moment on that tenuous tightrope can cause us to slip and lose our balance.

For millennia spiritual seekers found it necessary to retreat from the world. Whether they were taking refuge in the hills, caves, forests, or spiritual communities, the need for a safe haven was essential. This teaching advises us to seek balance, whether the temptation to veer from the state of equanimity comes from the material world or the celestial realm. Adhering to the path of balance, the yogi's pure heart rests exclusively with the Divine.

*Dwelling in a state of equanimity, the yogi neither accepts nor rejects admiration from others, even celestial beings; thus their heart stays pure and embraces only the Divine.*

III.53 *By* Samyama *on the smallest moment, as well as the succession of moments of time, the knowledge of supreme liberation is attained.*

By *Samyama* on the individual moment, the yogi realizes that the entire universe is transitory. When these moments are strung together, they form the phenomenon known as time. When holding on to time sequences, the thoughts, feelings, ideas, and actions venture from the past into the present moment. We then elicit projections of future happenings to join the mix and speculate on the outcomes. When the illusion of time is transcended, the knowledge of supreme liberation is gained.

This sutra reminds us that action can be forged or prevented only in the present moment, acknowledging the existing moment as the only reality. The past has gone with no hope of a do-over, and the future yet to come is anyone's guess.

As we are emancipated from the limits of time and space, the knowledge of supreme liberation is revealed.

**By** Samyama *on the smallest moment, as well as the succession of moments of time, the knowledge of supreme liberation is attained.*

## EXPERIENCING THE FLOW OF MOMENTS

*Sit in a comfortable meditative position.*

*Look at a clock and register the time as you begin this practice.*

*Allow the eyes to close and choosing an object begin to focus inward.*

*Observe how one solitary moment flows into the next.*

*When observed, do the moments slow down, speed up, or remain the same?*

*Are you able to assess each frame separately as an individual moment of time?*

*This is similar to the individual frames of a video, which, when viewed consecutively, form a moving documentary.*

*Begin to draw further inward, to the place where thought and feeling reside in the present moment.*

*Take in a deep breath and slowly allow the eyes to open.*

*Glance at the clock, and compare the time now to when you started.*

*Are you surprised? Was it a longer or shorter time than you expected?*

*If it seemed like one hour, and it was five minutes, you were still engaged with the thoughts.*

*If you gauged it to be five minutes and it was actually fifteen, you went beyond the constraints of time.*

*When time dissolves, the path to liberation is attainable.*

III.54 *With this exalted knowledge, the yogi is able to clearly distinguish even the most minute differences between two similar objects.*

III.55 *This intuitive knowledge, which has the ability to comprehend all objects under various conditions simultaneously, leads us to freedom.*

When the moments of time are transcended, the details that eluded us when perception was viewed in the confines of time are now discernible. They illuminate and focus our powers of discernment. We gain the ability to distinguish minute differences among various objects, either individually or as a whole.

When this comprehension activated by intuitive knowledge prevails, freedom manifests.

*With this exalted knowledge, the yogi is able to clearly distinguish even the most minute differences between two similar objects.*

*This intuitive knowledge, which has the ability to comprehend all objects under various conditions simultaneously, leads us to freedom.*

III.56 *Liberation is attained when the spiritual heart (Hridaya) attains purity equal to that of the True Self.*

After contemplating the powerful *siddhis* and assessing their attainability, we return full circle to the essence of *Hridaya,* the spiritual heart.

It is interesting to note that the words for "heart" in many traditions denote a multidimensional function for its expression, ultimately highlighting the essence of love and compassion.

The first aspect of heart is its function as a *physical* pump. The human heart, being the perfect servant, starts to circulate blood within weeks of conception and continues beating until the moment of physical death.

The second aspect of heart is the *emotional* heart. Saying "My heart is filled with love" or, conversely, "My heart is hurting" does not usually necessitate a trip to the emergency room. The expressions reflect an emotional aspect often attributed to the heart.

The third aspect of heart is *spiritual* or *Hridaya*. According to the Upanishads, *Hridaya* is "the dwelling place of the Self." Here the love and compassion the heart generates are ever ready and prepared for distribution. The *Hridaya* stays eternally pure.

The path of heart, while seemingly simple, is one to tread with sensitivity and care. Most spiritual traditions agree that the heart is the pathway to the Divine. A clear intellect, while prized, will only take us to the doorstep of liberation. To enter, we must place the *Hridaya* above all.

> Blessed are the pure in heart, for they shall see God.
>
> —*New Testament*

Follow your pure heart and it will lead you to your Divine Essence!

*Liberation is attained when the spiritual heart* (Hridaya) *attains purity equal to that of the True Self.*

# BOOK IV

# KAIVALYA PADA

## *Supreme Liberation*

"Kaivalya Pada: *Supreme Liberation*" begins by further expounding
on the attributes of the psychic and spiritual powers (siddhis). It
goes on to emphasize how it is necessary to transcend the gunas
(attributes of nature) in order to attain liberation, and it proclaims
the path of renunciation as the force that propels the yogi toward
knowing the freedom of the True Self.

Kaivalya Pada *then plunges into a valiant attempt to describe our
indescribable cosmic nature, which is beyond qualities or conditions.
Expanding into new dimensions, our consciousness recognizes
itself as a limitless and infinite spirit. Then the exalted yogi radiates
supreme wisdom, becoming a shining beacon of light living only to
serve humanity while maintaining the wisdom and radiance of the
Divine Self.*

# *SIDDHIS* AND POWER

*K*AIVALYA PADA ENTICES us toward liberation. The esoteric nature of this *pada* makes it clear that for liberation to occur, we must relinquish our former ideas of what and who we are. In their stead we embrace the wonderment that is awaiting us as we spiritually evolve. Through this transformation we become ensconced in the precious freedom, once envisioned as abstract, now within our reach.

> Siddhis (*powers*) *manifest through spiritual practices performed in previous births or through the use of herbs, mantra repetition, asceticism, or immersion in* Samadhi.

> *Due to the transforming power of spiritual practices, nature's energy flows with such abundance that it aids the spiritual seeker's evolution toward gaining a higher birth.*

> *While the practices do not directly affect transformation, they act to prevent obstacles from blocking the flow of nature's energy, needed for liberation.*

*Identification with the individual self (Asmita) creates the*
*chitta and its myriad thoughts and emotions.*

*Under certain conditions consciousness branches*
*into many different types of thoughts, feelings, or actions.*
*This is rooted in a mistaken sense of individuality*
*rather than the true source of oneness.*

IV.I Siddhis *(powers) manifest through spiritual practices performed in previous births or through the use of herbs, mantra repetition, asceticism, or immersion in* Samadhi.

At the very outset of *Kaivalya Pada,* we are offered ways to encourage the coveted *siddhis,* or powers, to manifest, exciting and tantalizing the practitioner. We become entranced by tales of superheroes or Yoga adepts capturing the attention of onlookers with their amazing feats.

In general, we are cautioned to allow this process to unfold naturally, yet the very first sutra suggests some aids to accompany us toward that fulfillment. While the use of herbs, chemicals, or austere practices may prompt a temporary state of "enlightenment," it remains as fragile as a thin ray of sunshine amid a stormy sky. Could it be that they are presented as an encouragement or perhaps to offer a taste of that coveted enlightenment? While they might aid in manifesting the powers initially, to sustain them requires deep and continuous spiritual practice. Often with temporary acquisition, the powers slowly dissipate, leaving just enough residue to delude us into believing we have reached enlightenment.

It might be difficult to know if the *siddhis* have ripened from a previous birth or from purity of heart. But does it really matter? Do the *siddhis* lie dormant within us? Can the right circumstances cause them to manifest?

Herbs have been used to heighten spiritual awareness for millennia. If administered under the close scrutiny of a mentor or spiritual teacher, the results can be insightful. There are also the forever curious who choose to experiment on their own, often with mixed results. Some may scale the summit of expanded consciousness, while others uncover a surge of disagreeable thoughts and feelings meant to remain dormant.

Drugs can never give you permanent higher wisdom. They can just
excite your mind a little, just like a strong dose of liquor. You may have
fantastic visions, but it is all within the mind—what is buried in the mind
is disturbed and thrown up to the surface. . . . Anything that is there
will be magnified, that is all. . . . All the impressions that are stored in the
mind are just pushed out; drugs cannot create a new impression or a new
idea and they can never bring the mind into a peaceful state.

—*Sri Swami Satchidananda*

Also encased in this sutra is the reference to mantra *japa,* or repetition of a word or sound. This practice is touted for our present
time period, the *Kali Yuga,* when spiritual consciousness is down-
graded as compared to other ages. During this time when the light
of truth is at its dimmest, even the smallest gesture, the repetition
of a sacred sound or mantra, can kindle the flame, increasing the
light.

Through deep awareness, the psychic powers, when gained, are
understood in proper perspective.

**Siddhis (***powers***) manifest through spiritual practices performed
in previous births or through the use of herbs, mantra
repetition, asceticism, or immersion in Samadhi.**

IV.2 *Due to the transforming power of spiritual
practices, nature's energy flows with such abundance
that it aids the spiritual seeker's evolution toward
gaining a higher birth.*

This is very encouraging! If we practice regularly and with zeal,
then nature's energy will flow with such abundance that it trans-

forms consciousness itself. Even our everyday life is impacted by this force of nature transforming the simplest action into a dynamic feat. The extraordinary now becomes the ordinary. By continual practice, this dynamic energy minimizes the restless thoughts and emotions, freeing us from the bonds of *Avidya*.

*Due to the transforming power of spiritual practices, nature's energy flows with such abundance that it aids the spiritual seeker's evolution toward gaining a higher birth.*

## IV.3 *While the practices do not directly affect transformation, they act to prevent obstacles from blocking the flow of nature's energy, needed for liberation.*

Regular practice plays an important role in preventing obstacles from diverting our focus from higher consciousness. To understand how the obstacles block the flow of energy, let's use the analogy of a simple plumbing issue.

In a functioning bathroom sink the water circles the drain before it disappears. When the smallest obstacle is present, even a few hairs, the downward flow of water is impeded. At first the movement of the water is merely reduced, but if the blockage is not remedied, it will cease to drain. Once the obstacle is removed, the force of gravity takes the lead, and the water drains smoothly.

Through continuous inward practice we gain the ability to alter the path of obstructive thoughts and emotions. When nature's energy is permitted to flow unencumbered, we move freely toward liberation.

*While the practices do not directly affect transformation, they act to prevent obstacles from blocking the flow of nature's energy, needed for liberation.*

IV.4 *Identification with the individual self (Asmita) creates the chitta and its myriad thoughts and emotions.*

IV.5 *Under certain conditions consciousness branches into many different types of thoughts, feelings, or actions. This is rooted in a mistaken sense of individuality rather than the true source of oneness.*

Here we again meet *Asmita,* one of the *Kleshas,* mistaking the individual self for the True Self. In the beginning stages of practice, this mistaken identification may not be evident. If our understanding erroneously designates the individual self and its actions as the source, the more subtle attributes of spiritual liberation are obscured from view.

One of the prime reasons to engage in continual spiritual practice is to spark the ability to discriminate between the individual self and the True Self. This is actualized by careful observation of behavioral patterns. If the energy needed for continued momentum can be diverted, all thought and emotion become weakened at their source, thus granting us mastery over the *chitta.*

As we continue to progress in our spiritual development, a deeper knowledge percolates through. Bestowed with even the smallest glimpse of our true nature, we are enticed inward, coaxing all awareness to withdraw from the external senses (*Pratyahara*).

The reward is the discovery of a world not even imagined, a vision that will forever change the way we see, feel, and experience who we really are.

*Identification with the individual self (Asmita) creates the* chitta *and its myriad thoughts and emotions.*

*Under certain conditions consciousness branches into many different types of thoughts, feelings, or actions. This is rooted in a mistaken sense of individuality rather than the true source of oneness.*

# THE POWER OF KARMA

K ARMA, THE HIDDEN force that influences all actions, is perceived as either good or bad. Our reaction to those actions and the obstacles they manifest is further expounded upon in these sutras. We are offered empowering alternatives to accepting karma as unchangeable.

*Through deep meditation the* chitta *becomes impotent and one becomes free from karma.*

*The actions (karmas) of the yogi, transformed through* **Dhyana,** *meditation, are neutralized and are therefore neither good nor bad, while the actions of others are still categorized as either good, bad, or mixed.*

*When those three types of actions (karmas) have favorable conditions, they create impressions that have the ability to manifest at any moment in time.*

*Because memory holds on to past impressions, the chain of cause and effect (karma) remains intact from one life to the next, as if there were no separation between births.*

*These past impressions are created without
beginning or end, fueling the perpetual cycle of
birth and death and the desire for immortality.*

*Impressions and desires that manifest because
of the veils covering the inner light (Kleshas) are
bound together by cause and effect. Resolving back into
seed form, they cease to function.*

IV.6 *Through deep meditation the* chitta *becomes impotent and one becomes free from karma.*

Depending on what type of karma is manifesting, it either hinders or facilitates the progress of our spiritual evolution. Upon entering a deep state of meditation (*Dhyana*), the *chitta* weakens, resulting in the release from karmic bonds.

The determination and tenacity it took to reach this exalted meditative state is now replaced with an effortless propulsion toward higher consciousness. As we continue to move deeper inward, any previous identification with the individual self (*Asmita*) is left behind.

We are then able to revitalize our sojourn toward liberation with minimal obstacles.

**Through deep meditation the** chitta **becomes impotent and one becomes free from karma.**

IV.7 *The actions (karmas) of the yogi, transformed through* Dhyana, *meditation, are neutralized and are therefore neither good nor bad, while the actions of others are still categorized as either good, bad, or mixed.*

For the yogi, the progression through *Dhyana* (deep meditation) renders all actions (karmas) neutral, absolving them from being categorized as either good or bad. In their neutrality the karmas are powerless to exert influence on our lives or the lives of others, while those who shy away from the quest for deeper knowledge still experience myriad thoughts and emotions categorized as good, bad, or mixed actions.

"Good" and "bad" are convenient terms to classify actions, but not necessarily accurate. Karma is inherently a neutral energy, neither good nor bad. The dual labels of "good" *or* "bad" are applied when an incident or action passes through the polarizing thoughts and emotions. Even in similar situations karma could be judged good in one instance, while the next time considered bad. If it vacillates between the two, it is identified as mixed, sometimes good, other times bad. Through *Dhyana,* karma is neutralized, and we are released from its bonds.

*The actions (karmas) of the yogi, transformed through* **Dhyana,** *meditation, are neutralized and are therefore neither good nor bad, while the actions of others are still categorized as either good, bad, or mixed.*

IV.8 *When those three types of actions (karmas) have favorable conditions, they create impressions that have the ability to manifest at any moment in time.*

We are cautioned that as long as we continue to identify with the three types of actions—good, bad, and mixed—we remain in worldly pursuits and under the jurisdiction of karma. It is through deep spiritual practice that karma is rendered powerless to create impressions and actions.

*When those three types of actions (karmas) have favorable conditions, they create impressions that have the ability to manifest at any moment in time.*

iv.9 *Because memory holds on to past impressions, the chain of cause and effect (karma) remains intact from one life to the next, as if there were no separation between births.*

Past impressions are held in the memory, explaining how an action not nullified continues to haunt our thoughts and emotions. Holding on to past impressions not only causes reactions but can manifest as actions that accompany us into the future and even into our next incarnation.

At age ninety my mother decided to delve into the mystical. Acquiring a book from a reputable seer of modern times, she called me for verification. "I read that if I do not make up with my sister and brother before I die, that I will be with them again in my next life," she said. "Do you believe that?"

"I do," I said with a bit of an inner smile.

"Well, then I will call them and make up right now! It is bad enough I had to endure them this life. The next one or future lives are not an option!"

The vast universe is a wheel upon which all creatures are subject to the cycle of birth death and rebirth. Round and round it turns and never stops. As long as the individual self perceives itself as separate from the Divine, it continues to revolve upon the wheel. But when through divine intervention it realizes they are one, it revolves upon the wheel no longer. It achieves immortality.

—Upanishads

*Because memory holds on to past impressions, the chain of cause and effect (karma) remains intact from one life to the next, as if there were no separation between births.*

## EXPERIENCING THE SEEDS OF KARMA

*Sit quietly, and inhale deeply as the body, thoughts, and emotions quiet.*

*Allow the mind to drift toward an incident or action that you perceive as unpleasant.*

*Form a full picture with all the emotions intact.*

*Begin to search for the cause of this action.*

*Can you find even the smallest seed of something you might have done, whether intentionally or unintentionally, that could have caused this type of action?*

*Perhaps you spoke an unkind word in a moment of anger or caused pain to another that is now returning as an action to diminish your peace.*

*Once the action has been launched, the only thing we have control over is our reaction to it.*

*Begin to project a positive attitude toward the people involved.*

*Experience a state of inner calmness and know the correct remedy for many wrongdoings is forgiveness and acceptance.*

*These can be applied whether or not you have inadvertently caused the regretful action.*

IV.10 *These past impressions are created without beginning or end, fueling the perpetual cycle of birth and death and the desire for immortality.*

IV.11 *Impressions and desires that manifest because of the veils covering the inner light (Kleshas) are bound together by cause and effect. Resolving back into seed form, they cease to function.*

The obstacles, or *Kleshas,* explained in sutra II.3 (page 128) are referred to in subsequent sutras, as they form major impediments to our liberation. No matter how dim it is, if we focus on the inner light for guidance, any doubts and fears entrenched in the *Kleshas* can be released. By concealing the inner light, our true nature is thwarted.

The *Kleshas* are continually reintroduced in the sutras due to their importance in understanding the pathway to freedom. The primary *Klesha, Avidya,* innocence of our divine nature, is the one that creates the fertile field for the seeds of the other *Kleshas* to manifest. When we gain discernment, the impediments responsible for the perpetual cycle of birth and death can be resolved back into seed form.

As we begin to comprehend the impact these obstacles have on our path to liberation, the Yoga Sutras graciously offer methods to dissolve them. Once the *Kleshas* have manifested into words or actions, they have deeply rooted. Mere observation is not enough to displace them. This is the time to call upon the deeper, subtler, and therefore more powerful inner practices. Periods of stillness, introspection, and devotion are summoned to dissolve the veils that hide the inner light.

*These past impressions are created without beginning or end, fueling the perpetual cycle of birth and death and the desire for immortality.*

*Impressions and desires that manifest because of the veils covering the inner light (Kleshas) are bound together by cause and effect. Resolving back into seed form, they cease to function.*

# THE PLAY OF THE *GUNAS*

HERE THE THREE *gunas* (attributes of nature) are distinguished as hindrances to our ultimate liberation. They influence our perception, distracting us from recognizing obstacles on our path. Harnessing their movements transports us toward realization of the True Self.

*Both past and future simultaneously exist in all objects,*
*while exhibiting different characteristics*
*due to the movements of nature (gunas).*

*Past, present, and future, whether manifested or subtle, are*
*caused by fluctuation of the gunas.*

*When they are unbalanced, the play of the gunas causes*
*modifications in an object, but if they are in balance, the*
*unique essence and expression of the object do not change.*

*Due to differences in understanding and the various ways one*
*perceives objects and actions, each person may view the same*
*object differently, according to their own perception.*

*Therefore, the object is not dependent on a single perception.*
*Otherwise, the object would be said to be nonexistent if that*
*one individual is not perceiving it.*

*The essence of an object is known or unknown
according to the conditioning or expectation of
the individual consciousness perceiving it.*

*The Seer, being omniscient, observes the changes and
transformations taking place within the thoughts and emotions.*

IV.12 *Both past and future simultaneously exist in all objects, while exhibiting different characteristics due to the movements of nature* (gunas).

Time presents as the sequential relationship of one event to another and then that event to another and so on. We perceive this relationship as past, present, or future. Past incidents may merge into the present, *or* future projections might steal time from the present.

The movement of time exhibits different characteristics, fostering the illusion of the progression of time. Through our projections every incident either *has happened* or *will happen*.

Imagine yourself in a garden (present) observing a mature plant laden with ripe tomatoes sprouted from seeds planted last spring (past). The future intervenes as you project the many uses for the succulent fruit. All three points in the time sequence are present while observing the one plant.

It is through the movements of the *gunas* that the mind modifies time sequences and characteristics. When the mind and the *gunas* are no longer in play, the past and future weave together to form the ever-present *now*.

*Both past and future simultaneously exist in all objects, while exhibiting different characteristics due to the movements of nature* (gunas).

IV.13 *Past, present, and future, whether manifested or subtle, are caused by fluctuation of the* gunas.

Due to the play of the *gunas,* conditions continually change, creating the illusion that time has changed.

Time does not exist—we invented it. Time is what the clock says. The
distinction between the past, present and future is only a stubbornly
persistent illusion.

—*Albert Einstein*

*Past, present, and future, whether manifested or subtle, are
caused by fluctuation of the* gunas.

The forms and expressions of an object *may appear* to be new or
changed, yet they have always existed and will continue to exist
within the object. It seems to coincide with the scientific principle
that matter can be neither created nor destroyed.

The Bhagavad Gita explains this concept: "That which is nonexistent can never come into being, and that which is, can never
cease to be."

IV.14 *When they are unbalanced, the play of the* gunas
*cause modifications in an object, but if they are in
balance, the unique essence and expression of the object
does not change.*

IV.15 *Due to differences in understanding and the
various ways one perceives objects and actions, each
person may view the same object differently, according
to their own perception.*

IV.16 *Therefore, the object is not dependent on a single perception. Otherwise, the object would be said to be nonexistent if that one individual is not perceiving it.*

This concept can be understood by observing the changes in our daily lives. When we are happy, we project that all are happy. If we feel unhappy, we assume that most are unhappy. Before we are able to embrace the concept of oneness, we perceive the world through the lens of *our* desires and prejudices. Even Marie Antoinette, when told that the people were starving from lack of bread, based her evaluation on her own larder. Well, she said, if they do not have enough bread to stave off their hunger, let them eat brioche instead. She concluded that if the sweet bread was available to her, it must be so for everyone.

The question of perception is found in many wisdom teachings and is reminiscent of the well-known Zen koan "If a tree falls in the forest and there is no one to hear it, does it make a sound?" This has caused many a student of Buddhism to ponder the nature of existence and their role in it.

If we can hear it, smell it, taste it, see it, does that make it real? Does it appear real to everyone, or is reality dependent on the senses of the perceiver? This sutra advises us that an object's existence is not dependent on any single perception.

*Due to differences in understanding and the various ways one perceives objects and actions, each person may view the same object differently, according to their own perception.*

*Therefore, the object is not dependent on a single perception. Otherwise, the object would be said to be nonexistent if that one individual is not perceiving it.*

iv.17 *The essence of an object is known or unknown according to the conditioning or expectation of the individual consciousness perceiving it.*

Here we are reminded that when an object is viewed by a variety of people, it appears different according to their experiences. Our point of reference and identification are based on past impressions and future expectations.

It is similar to the parable about three blindfolded people describing an elephant based on touch. The person feeling the tail would describe the elephant as a rope. To the one touching the leg, it feels like a tree trunk. If the ear is the object of inspection, it could be labeled as a fan. Each person is convinced that they have the complete picture of how the elephant appears, forgetting it is based on their limited experience. It is their distorted perception that causes them to doubt other conclusions *and* the totality of the elephant.

Discerning an object with our limited sensory input, we are privy to only a small part of the whole situation. As the power of introspection develops, our previous conditioning and expectations expand exponentially. We then understand that our individual insight is only one aspect of any given situation.

*The essence of an object is known or unknown according to the conditioning or expectation of the individual consciousness perceiving it.*

## IV.18 *The Seer, being omniscient, observes the changes and transformations taking place within the thoughts and emotions.*

It would be a great boon to gain insight into our mental processes and to easily change them. Our way of perceiving objects and life as a whole would be greatly altered. There is an interesting concept in Yoga wisdom that suggests that the mind, with its myriad thoughts and emotions, projects outward as color (*varna*). Perceiving the vibrational color of the mind activates all the senses, not only sight. When we identify the projections of the mind as color (*varna*), much of the judgment can be released. We gain the ability to influence the way thoughts and emotions are both projected *and* received. If thoughts and emotions are identified as color, changing the mental outlook could be as simple as altering the hue.

Even without realizing it, we are already assigning color to our thoughts and emotions. When we say, "I feel *blue* today," we are letting others know that we are a bit unhappy, not that we actually appear as the color blue. We might say someone is *green* with envy, *red* with rage, and so on. Those of us who happen to remain cheery through life's trials and tribulations are often accused of looking at the world through *rose*-colored glasses. Not being deterred by others' opinions, we tend to see the rosy side of life.

Although the color reflected by the mind does not actually affect our physical appearance, we have to wonder how it affects the radiance of our auric field.

Recognizing that the thoughts and emotions radiate color, by changing the color, we change their effect!

*The Seer, being omniscient, observes the changes and transformations taking place within the thoughts and emotions.*

## EXPERIENCING THE EFFECT OF THOUGHTS AND EMOTIONS AS COLOR

*Sit comfortably, take in a few deep breaths, and let them out slowly.*

*Choose a dominant thought or emotion that is expressing itself right now.*

*Observe the expression and notice if you can detect even a hint of color that it might be emitting.*

*If it seems to be devoid of color, choose any hue to infuse into it.*

*Notice if it accepts or rejects the color. If the color is rejected, try another shade.*

*Continue going through the color wheel until you find one that conveys what you are experiencing.*

*If the thought is vibrating as green, and that does not suit you, try changing it to another color, for example, pink. If that does not feel right, try red or sunny yellow.*

*Take in a few deep breaths. Breathe in all the colors of the rainbow.*

*The more you experiment with colors, the more accessible they will become and the easier it will be to create the vibration of your choosing.*

# THE *CHITTA*, THE SENSES, AND THE TRUE SELF

THE SENSES ARE vital for keeping ourselves safe and enjoying all the wonders of the outer world. But in doing so we become rooted in the material. In order for us to traverse the subtle, the senses must oblige and turn inward.

*Knowledge and perception can be experienced only by the Seer, as the* chitta *is not self-luminous.*

*Without the inner light, the* chitta *is unable to perceive both subject and object simultaneously.*

*The various thoughts and feelings contained in the* chitta *are reflections of a single consciousness that is all-knowing and unchangeable.*

*When pure consciousness illuminates the* chitta, *it simulates the reflections and characteristics of that consciousness, causing the* chitta *to appear conscious.*

*The* chitta, *in order to distinguish an object of perception, must assume knowledge from the one consciousness.*

*Though having countless desires, the* chitta *seeks not only to satisfy the senses but also to further the emancipation of the soul.*

IV.19 *Knowledge and perception can be experienced only by the Seer, as the* chitta *is not self-luminous.*

The Seer, being self-effulgent like the sun, has the ability to shine light and illumine objects. Neither the *chitta* nor the objects themselves have the capacity to project light. They can be compared to a mirror that reflects rather than being the source of the illumination. Once the self-effulgent light of the True Self that dwells within our hearts is revealed, it radiates outward, illuminating all objects, animate or inanimate.

*Knowledge and perception can be experienced only by the Seer, as the* chitta *is not self-luminous.*

IV.20 *Without the inner light, the* chitta *is unable to perceive both subject and object simultaneously.*

The sun shines of its own accord, but the moon's luminosity is simply a reflection of the sun. Similarly, the soul/Seer is self-illumined but not the *chitta* (individual consciousness). When the various spheres of *chitta* are vividly perceived during different states of *Samadhi,* it then becomes the subject, rather than the object, of perception and knowledge. The moment the *chitta* has the ability to observe itself, it transcends the limits of the thoughts, feelings, and senses. The *chitta* is now like the moon, reflecting the light of the True Self.

*Without the inner light, the* chitta *is unable to perceive both subject and object simultaneously.*

IV.21 *The various thoughts and feelings contained in the* chitta *are reflections of a single consciousness that is all-knowing and unchangeable.*

IV.22 *When pure consciousness illuminates the* chitta, *it simulates the reflections and characteristics of that consciousness, causing the* chitta *to appear conscious.*

IV.23 *The* chitta, *in order to distinguish an object of perception, must assume knowledge from the one consciousness.*

Imagine there are satellite clusters of thoughts and emotions stemming from the *chitta*. These clusters of similar thoughts and emotions have grouped together for a purpose. One cluster may be concerned with health and self-care, while another may be in opposition, making unhealthy choices. The farther the clusters stray from their essential nature, the more inconsistent and unfocused they become, creating erratic thinking, personalities, and moods. The inconsistent focus makes it difficult to garner a single purpose. An illusion of independence manifests when the *chitta* perceives the thoughts and emotions as comprehensive, rather than a small and often fragmented reflection of consciousness.

Faced with a decision, we may say, "My heart says one thing, but my mind wants another." It is as if the *chitta* is dividing itself into multiple aspects, seeking either the same or different outcomes. When different options loom, the division between heart and head makes reaching a decisive conclusion difficult. If *only* the *chitta* is recognized, one is unable to reach the discernment necessary to distinguish the movements of consciousness. At other times, the pure consciousness remains the source of wisdom.

*The various thoughts and feelings contained in the* chitta *are reflections of a single consciousness that is all-knowing and unchangeable.*

*When pure consciousness illuminates the* chitta, *it simulates the reflections and characteristics of that consciousness, causing the* chitta *to appear conscious.*

*The* chitta, *in order to distinguish an object of perception, must assume knowledge from the one consciousness.*

## EXPERIENCING THE REUNION OF THE *CHITTA*

*Sit comfortably, take in a few deep breaths, and let them out slowly.*

*Begin to observe the thoughts and emotions.*

*Reach into the near or distant past and bring forth a memory of a decision you made.*

*Look at it as if it were new.*

*Try to recall what the dilemma was and how it was resolved.*

*Was it the mind's logic or the heart's compassion that won?*

*From a place of elevated consciousness, observe which solution (logic or compassion) resonates more closely with your nature.*

*Did the resolution you made solve this issue?*

*As you inhale, allow the mind and heart to open to other possibilities.*

*Exhale, allowing doubts to dissipate.*

*If new possibilities surfaced, project them onto the situation until the negative feelings subside.*

*If it is a situation you frequently encounter, repeat this practice as often as possible and be amazed at the changes.*

*Take in a few breaths and return to the present.*

*Keep remembering that by resolving the consciousness back to the heart, we remain entwined with the Divine.*

**IV.24** *Though having countless desires, the* chitta *seeks not only to satisfy the senses but also to further the emancipation of the soul.*

As we evolve, even the *chitta* that was assumed to be satisfied with the play of *Maya* (illusion) seeks liberation. While desires are still present, they become less and less seductive. It can be likened to a child who has been given many toys to entice her, but their attraction fails when a sweet puppy enters the room. All that had occupied the youngster's time and affection is suddenly dwarfed when a living playmate arrives in her world.

Once the possibility of freedom is accorded to us, all desires, large and small, seem like bondage when compared to the great liberation.

*Though having countless desires, the* chitta *seeks not only to satisfy the senses but also to further the emancipation of the soul.*

# DISCRIMINATION

CONTINUOUS DISCRIMINATION IS necessary in order for elevated consciousness to touch every aspect of our daily lives. When this discrimination is fostered not only in the formal practices but in every aspect of existence, the liberation we crave is realized.

*By increased discrimination, the* chitta *ceases to identify itself as the Divine Consciousness.*

*Then the* chitta, *enticed toward discrimination, propels itself toward liberation.*

*If discrimination becomes lax, distractions due to past impressions may arise.*

*These distractions from enlightenment can be redirected through inward practices in the same manner as we dissolve the veils over the inner light, the Kleshas.*

IV.25 *By increased discrimination, the* chitta *ceases to identify itself as the Divine Consciousness.*

Here we begin to understand the necessity of fielding discrimination throughout the day. Our formal meditation practice gives us insights and hones discrimination. But it is the issues that assault us daily that become perfect fodder for expanding the understanding that has been revealed during *Dhyana*.

When the clarity that we are not the *chitta* coalesces, we no longer identify ordinary thoughts and feelings as divine guidance. It becomes clear which stem from the mind and which emanate from the source. If we relegate our discrimination to only formal practices, the full impact of this identity with the Divine Consciousness is denied.

**By increased discrimination, the chitta ceases to identify itself as the Divine Consciousness.**

IV.26 *Then the* chitta, *enticed toward discrimination, propels itself into liberation.*

Once the *chitta* gains this realization, it is catapulted toward liberation. Why should it settle for a reflection of the Divine Self when it can become the source?

Consider that for most seekers the Self exists only in theory, so when it is finally glimpsed, we are rapidly drawn to it. It is similar to walking into a darkened room in your home, unable to see objects due to the lack of light. With the flick of a switch, you now easily see what could not be perceived in darkness.

The *chitta,* positioned between consciousness and the external objects it powers, is like the darkened room. Unable to radiate light, it cannot recognize itself as an object. It remains a *reflection* of the light of Divine Consciousness.

*Then the* chitta, *enticed toward discrimination, propels itself into liberation.*

## iv.27 *If discrimination becomes lax, distractions due to past impressions may arise.*

Here we are encouraged to be constantly discriminating, both in our formal practices and in daily life. It is the hope that by elevating consciousness, our discriminative abilities become steady. That is why we are cautioned that becoming lax in discernment distracts us from the path of liberation. If we forget the power and tenacity of past impressions, they gain the ability to reestablish themselves in our thoughts and emotions, thus causing us to once again forget our true nature.

*If discrimination becomes lax, distractions due to past impressions may arise.*

## iv.28 *These distractions from enlightenment can be redirected through inward practices in the same manner as we dissolve the veils over the inner light, the* Kleshas.

Spirit and nature are unable to bind together because of *Avidya* (the absence of knowledge). It is the *Kleshas,* or the five veils covering the light of the Divine Self, that obscure it from recognition.

The remedy for this is to plunge deeply into the subtle aspects of our spiritual quest, including *Samadhi* and *Samyama*. These elevated states grant us the power to dispel any distraction.

Through the deeper states our awareness is enhanced, and nature's hold on us lessens. As one by one the veils dissipate, the divine light within is seen again. The moment we turn toward the light, we are welcomed, and liberation becomes a reality.

*These distractions from enlightenment can be redirected through inward practices in the same manner as we dissolve the veils over the inner light, the* Kleshas.

6

# SUPREME LIBERATION

HERE WE RELEASE the final hold on any distractions to our enlightenment. Remembering our true nature, we are obliged to live an exalted and conscious life. Realizing these truths, we are propelled into supreme liberation.

*Through the grace of Intuitive Wisdom, one remains totally disinterested even in the possession of all the psychic powers and ascends to the Cloud of Virtue (Dharmamegha Samadhi).*

*Reaching the exalted state of Dharmamegha Samadhi (the Cloud of Virtue), all sufferings and karmas cease.*

*Upon realization of this infinite knowledge, the entire universe, with all its sense objects, loses its powers of attraction.*

*The gunas, having fulfilled their purpose, become impotent.*

*In the final stages of liberation, the fluctuation of the gunas ceases to function, causing time to become irrelevant.*

*Kaivalya, liberation, manifests as the impotent gunas reabsorb themselves into Prakriti (nature), revealing the exalted consciousness shining forth as Divine Light.*

IV.29 *Through the grace of Intuitive Wisdom, one remains totally disinterested even in the possession of all the psychic powers and ascends to the Cloud of Virtue* (Dharmamegha Samadhi).

When a high level of consciousness is achieved, the yogi realizes the *siddhis* are a hindrance to enlightenment and becomes disinterested in pursuing them further. The only aspirations that still remain are to sustain spiritual connection, to be compassionate, and to live forever in unsurpassed bliss. We often imagine that when this state is reached, withdrawal from the world is imminent, yet it is possible to live and serve in the world while maintaining an elevated consciousness.

> Keep the hand in society, while the heart rests with the Divine.
> —Bhagavad Gita

*Through the grace of Intuitive Wisdom, one remains totally disinterested even in the possession of all the psychic powers and ascends to the Cloud of Virtue* (**Dharmamegha Samadhi**).

IV.30 *Reaching the exalted state of* Dharmamegha Samadhi *(the Cloud of Virtue), all sufferings and karmas cease.*

It is important to understand what is meant by suffering. When an incident or accident occurs, there are many aspects at play. One is physical pain. Having experienced any type of strong physical pain, we know that it feels *very real*. If the pain persists over a long period of time, it tends to drain any and all available energy. It is so debilitating that there are specialties in medicine just to assist in the management and treatment of chronic physical pain.

The companion to the physical pain is a bit more difficult to comprehend and successfully treat. When the physical pain enlists the emotions, it becomes *suffering*. Initially for most, it is difficult to separate the physical pain from the emotional suffering. After some time, the physical pain may subside, but that is not always the case with suffering. Months or even years after the physical pain has retreated, if we reunite with the memory of the incident, the suffering can easily resurface.

We must acknowledge and treat our emotional suffering with deep compassion. Otherwise, mental anguish will accumulate in the memory, reasserting itself when the climate is right. It could reoccur while anticipating an unpleasant event or become reinvigorated through another injury or illness. When we hitch our consciousness to the star of enlightenment and liberation, all sufferings cease.

*Reaching the exalted state of* Dharmamegha Samadhi *(the Cloud of Virtue), all sufferings and karmas cease.*

## IV.31 *Upon realization of this infinite knowledge, the entire universe, with all its sense objects, loses its powers of attraction.*

Staying anchored to the path of higher consciousness even when psychic powers beckon, the yogi is granted all the knowledge in the universe. It showers a "cloud of virtue" upon us, bestowing liberation and the bliss of Divine Consciousness.

It was a beautiful day as we landed in San José, Costa Rica. This was my second visit to this unique country, which possesses multiple diverse ecosystems.

Leading a retreat on the opposite side of the country necessitated going over a treacherous mountain pass. The natives called it the Cloud Forest. I quickly understood the reason for the name as we began our ascent.

Just the idea of driving up into a cloud and allowing it to surround me seemed quite mystical, and I was hoping for an ethereal experience. As we gained altitude, the mist started to envelop us.

At a certain point we could no longer see the road or the lines painted on it. The sense of excitement dwindled in direct proportion to our ability to see our surroundings. I tried in vain to look outside, but the visibility was totally obliterated. Whether I looked to the side, front, or rear, only clouds and nothingness surrounded me. My senses seem to have hushed; none were giving their customary feedback. It was as if they also had retreated into the clouds. I felt myself going into another dimension where there was no future, no projection of what could be. My thoughts and emotions were being reoriented to make this harrowing adventure into an amusing exploration. The only choice I had was to be in the present moment, nestled in a cloud. Somehow not projecting into the future or looking into the past allowed me a deep sense of peace.

If we remain fixed to the past, it whisks us away from the present. When we project into the future, there are fewer possibilities for spontaneous changes to occur and more occasion for disappointment. Even as the clouds retreated on our descent, the cherished experience of existing solely in the present moment remained.

The Cloud Forest was a natural occurrence, but to me it became a spiritual lesson. Relishing the insight that both the past and present are illusions, our only choice is to live in the present moment.

*Upon realization of this infinite knowledge, the entire universe, with all its sense objects, loses its powers of attraction.*

IV.32 *The* gunas, *having fulfilled their purpose, become impotent.*

IV.33 *In the final stages of liberation, the fluctuation of the* gunas *ceases to function, causing time to become irrelevant.*

Our world is formed through the imbalance of the three aspects of nature, the *gunas* (*Sattwa, Rajas,* and *Tamas*), so that we may fully experience all its glories *and* sorrows. Ultimately, as consciousness expands, we tire of the constant tossing between pleasure and pain, right and wrong, all the dualities. Renouncing all worldly attachments becomes our only option for liberation. When liberation is bestowed, the *gunas* become impotent; their purpose has been fulfilled.

Anchoring to the ever-present moment, the omnipresent yogi experiences everything as occurring *now.* The past and future merge into the present moment, where all knowledge and wisdom reside—we then know everything.

*The* gunas, *having fulfilled their purpose, become impotent.*

*In the final stages of liberation, the fluctuation of the* gunas *ceases to function, causing time to become irrelevant.*

IV.34 Kaivalya, *liberation, manifests as the impotent* gunas *reabsorb themselves into* Prakriti *(nature), revealing the exalted consciousness shining forth as Divine Light.*

On arriving at the final sutra, we are infused with the knowledge that when renouncing the world of duality, we merge into the light of our own divine nature.

Then the kind and thoughtful nature goes back the same way it came, to retrieve others who also have lost their way in the trackless desert of life. Nature continues to create experiences of pleasure and pain, good and evil, until those who remained to fulfill their hopes and dreams are ready to ascend, while the yogis who have soared beyond duality join the infinite river of souls flowing into the ocean of oneness, attaining supreme liberation.

> Nature's task is done, this unselfish task which our sweet nurse,
> in the form of nature, has imposed upon itself. Gently taking
> the self-forgetting soul by the hand as it were and shows it all
> the experiences in the universe, all manifestations bringing
> it higher and higher through the various bodies, till its lost
> glory comes back and it remembers its own nature.
> —*Swami Vivekananda*

**Kaivalya, *liberation, manifests as the impotent* gunas *reabsorb themselves into* Prakriti (*nature*), *revealing the exalted consciousness shining forth as Divine Light.***

## EXPERIENCING MEDITATION ON THE DIVINE LIGHT IN US ALL

*Allow the body and mind to become quiet, and close the eyes.*

*Bring the awareness to the crown of the head, where there is a brilliant light of a thousand suns.*

*Through this portal observe as light streams in from a distant source, transforming the top of the head into light.*

*Take in a deep breath, and notice how the light brightens.*

*Exhale, sending that light out to the world.*

*Continue to follow the Divine Light as it moves outward through rivers and streams, oceans, cities and towns, embracing every living thing with light and love.*

*Inhale, and the light brightens.*

*Exhale, forming a circle of Divine Light surrounding the entire earth, encompassing all beings so that they may experience the light of their own divine nature.*

*As you inhale, the light brightens. With the exhale, send light and love out to the world.*

*Through this one light, all are united.*

*Affirm that the same light that shines within us shines in all. We are one in the light!*

**Glory unto those who have realized their own nature! May their blessings be on us all!**

# CONTINUING OUR LIFELONG STUDY
## OF THE YOGA SUTRAS

Having journeyed together through the Yoga Sutras, we now recognize Yoga as an essential *experiential wisdom* rather than a set of practices or a philosophy. With continued practice and experience, this extremely potent wisdom directs us like a compass to our magnetic divine nature.

Our wisdom compass has now brought us not just full circle but in an upward spiral, enabling us to revisit the foundational wisdom of the Yoga Sutras with a whole new understanding and insight. Each time we begin the study of the Yoga Sutras anew, we understand more profoundly—with our hearts—the ever-powerful wisdom they impart.

I myself delved yet again into the sutras to write this book, so that I could express them genuinely from my heart. This process required of me a great deal of faith and devotion. I would recall the many years of sitting with my guru, Sri Swami Satchidanandaji, as he expounded on the meaning of the sutras. I prayed often to the spirits of the goddesses, gods, gurus, saints, and sages to be elevated to Golden Age consciousness and understanding. Many graciously obliged my prayers. But amazingly, it was Sri Patanjali himself, the sage who first compiled the Yoga Sutras, who boosted me into a deeper realm of wisdom.

Moving about one of the great temples in South India, paying homage to the many resident goddesses and gods, I was drawn to a small shrine dedicated to "the perfect servant of the Divine," Sri Hanuman, housed in a far-removed area of the temple. Meditating at this shrine, I lost awareness of the physical realm.

Returning to the material plane, I followed the usual custom of circumambulating the shrine. My companions walked at a normal pace; I lagged behind them slightly.

Rounding the final corner of the shrine, I noticed that the sides of the temple were devoid of decoration or representation. I felt a "wall of energy" that seemed to physically halt me.

At once an "energy vortex" emanating from the blank stone wall drew me to it. When my eyes were able to focus, I saw a tiny oil lamp glowing behind a small, unmarked, soot-covered glass door.

By then my husband and friends had noticed that I was not with them, and they came back to find me, accompanied by a local priest. They seemed not to notice the "energy wall."

"That," said the priest to me, gesturing to the small shrine, "is the *Maha Samadhi* Shrine of Sri Patanjali, the final resting place of his remains."

I stayed transfixed on the spot, and my breathing ceased. After I had meditated on what Sri Patanjali could have said, thought, and meant for so many years, he had called me to him, bestowing the blessings of a Divine Being known as *darshan*.

What profound and direct message was he imparting to me? What essence of the Yoga Sutras did he divulge to me without spoken words? This will remain a mystery, a deep secret known only by my heart. I am grateful to have been blessed by Sri Patanjali and the countless others in a multitude of ways, and I pray that what I have expressed in this book reflects the truth of that blessed sanction.

For most of you, the study of Yoga will probably not extend to a pilgrimage to India, or to a lengthy period of study with a realized guru. But if you take what you have experienced in your Yoga practice and bring it into your life, you will find your life greatly improves.

Read the sutras; meditate on them; experience their true meaning. If you do this with your heart, you will know newfound enrichment in your Yoga practice, and in everything you do.

May we live in love and joy, knowing our own divine nature.

*Nischala Joy Devi*

# FOR FURTHER REFLECTION:
## THE YOGA SUTRAS
### HEARTFULLY EXPRESSED

This section is a listing of the sutras without commentary. They can be recited or written at any time and are especially powerful as a prelude to meditation. Reading the sutras is a meditative practice of its own.

It is beneficial to reflect on the flow of the Yoga Sutras and the way each sets the stage for the next, allowing the meaning of all the sutras to be understood with the heart. Reciting them as one continuum allows the essence of the sutras to be conveyed and discovered. *Sravana* (listening) is facilitated by repeating the sutra first aloud, then in a whisper, and finally with only the silence of the heart. This repetition in sequence honors the rhythm of the words and leads us to an understanding greater than each one could elicit individually.

Take a moment to draw in a deep breath and, with wholehearted awareness, repeat these sutras as you *listen* to the great teaching reverberating through your body, mind, emotions, and spirit. Allow the wisdom to be imparted. In this way you will access the deeper, more intuitive form of knowing. May you realize the joy that is your birthright.

I.1    With humility (an open heart and mind), we embrace the sacred study of Yoga.

I.2    Yoga is the uniting of consciousness in the heart.

I.3    United in the heart, consciousness is steadied, then we abide in our true nature—joy.

I.4    At other times, we identify with the rays of consciousness, which fluctuate and encourage our perceived suffering.

I.5    Dividing into five, these rays of consciousness polarize as pleasant or unpleasant.

I.6    The rays manifest as knowledge, misunderstanding, imagination, deep sleep, and memory.

I.7    *Knowledge* embraces personal experience, inference, and insights from the wise.

I.8    *Misunderstanding* comes when perception is unclear or tinted.

I.9    *Imagination* is kindled by hearing words, seeing images, or experiencing feelings.

I.10   *Deep sleep* allows us to withdraw from conscious awareness.

I.11   *Memory* is when a previous experience returns to conscious awareness.

I.12   Consciousness is elevated by *Abhyasa* (devoted practice) and *Vairagya* (remembering the Self).

I.13   Devoted practice, *Abhyasa*, cultivates the unfolding of consciousness.

I.14   *Abhyasa* is nurtured by a sustained, steady rhythm and a dedicated heart.

I.15   With constant remembrance of the Self, *Vairagya*, all yearnings fade.

I.16  When consciousness unites, it remains clear and unaffected by the external changes of nature, the *gunas*. This is the ultimate *Vairagya*.

I.17  By cultivation of *Abhyasa* and *Vairagya*, the intellect becomes keen, reasoning is clear, bliss is reflected to all, and outward identification unites with the Supreme Consciousness.

I.18  With continued awareness, we identify only with the pure consciousness residing in the heart.

I.19  Through identification with pure consciousness, the physical world can be transcended.

I.20  This identification is enhanced by faith, dynamism, intention, reflection, and perception.

I.21  To the dedicated and devoted, the divine truth is revealed.

I.22  Spiritual consciousness develops in direct proportion to one's dedication.

I.23  Boundless love and devotion unite us with the Divine Consciousness.

I.24  The Divine Consciousness is self-effulgent like the sun.

I.25  The Divine is the essence of all knowledge, wisdom, and love.

I.26  Knowledge, wisdom, and love are the omnipresent teachers, in all beings.

I.27  Repeating the sacred sound manifests Divine Consciousness.

I.28  When expressed with great devotion, the sacred sound reveals our divine nature.

I.29  By faithful repetition, the inner light luminously shines.

1.30            Perception of our true nature is often obscured by
                physical, mental, and emotional imbalances.

1.31            These imbalances can promote restlessness, uneven
                breathing, worry, and loss of hope.

1.32            These imbalances can be prevented from engaging by
                developing loyalty to a sacred practice.

1.33            To preserve openness of heart and calmness of mind,
                nurture these attitudes:

                    *Kindness to those who are happy*

                    *Compassion for those who are less fortunate*

                    *Honor for those who embody noble qualities*

                    *Equanimity to those whose actions oppose your values*

1.34            Slow, easeful exhalations can be used to restore and
                preserve balance.

1.35            Or engage the focus on an inspiring object.

1.36            Or cultivate devotion to the supreme, ever-blissful light
                within.

1.37            Or receive grace from a great soul who exudes divine
                qualities.

1.38            Or reflect on a peaceful feeling from an experience, a
                dream, or deep sleep.

1.39            Or dedicate yourself to anything that elevates and
                embraces your heart.

1.40            Gradually through focused awareness one's knowledge
                extends from the smallest atom to the greatest
                magnitude.

1.41            As a naturally pure crystal appears to take the color
                of everything around it yet remains unchanged,
                the yogi's heart remains pure and unaffected by its

surroundings while attaining a state of oneness with all. This is *Samadhi*.

1.42    When awareness merges with a "material" object or form, if the *name, quality,* and *knowledge* are perceived, this is *Savitarka Samadhi,* or reflective *Samadhi*.

1.43    When awareness merges with a "material" object or form, if *knowledge alone* is perceived, this is *Nirvitarka Samadhi,* or spontaneous *Samadhi*.

1.44    When awareness merges with a "subtle" object or form, two different *Samadhis* are present, *Savichara* (perceiving *name, quality,* and *knowledge*) and *Nirvichara* (perceiving *knowledge alone*).

1.45    These states of *Samadhi* have the power to extend beyond all the "material" and "subtle" forms and objects, to reveal nature in her unmanifested form.

1.46    All the *Samadhis* described thus far have been *Sabija* (with seed), which have the ability to germinate, returning us to ordinary consciousness.

1.47    In the purity of *Nirvichara Samadhi,* Divine Consciousness becomes luminescent.

1.48    When consciousness dwells in *absolute, true knowledge* (*Ritambhara Prajna*), direct spiritual perception dawns.

1.49    This *absolute, true knowledge* (*Ritambhara Prajna*) is totally different from the knowledge gained by personal experience, inference, and insights from the wise.

1.50    When experiencing this *absolute, true knowledge* (*Ritambhara Prajna*), all previous *Samskaras* (impressions) are left behind and new ones are prevented from sprouting.

I.51        *Nirbija* (seedless) *Samadhi* outshines all impressions
            and manifestations.

II.1        *Kriya Yoga,* or Yoga in action, embraces:

            *Tapas:* igniting the purifying flame

            *Swadhaya:* sacred study of the Divine through
            scripture, nature, and introspection

            *Iswara Pranidhana:* wholehearted dedication to the
            Divine Light in all

II.2        These practices enhance inner awareness and guide us
            to liberation.

II.3        Dissolving the five *Kleshas,* or veils, brings forth the
            radiance of the Divine Self.

            The five *Kleshas,* or veils, are:

            *Avidya:* innocence of our divine nature

            *Asmita:* undue trust in the individual self

            *Raga:* excessive fondness for fleeting pleasures

            *Dvesa:* excessive avoidance of unpleasant
            experiences

            *Abhinivesah:* elusive awareness of immortality

II.4        Innocence of our divine nature (*Avidya*) creates a
            fertile field where the dormant seeds of the other
            four veils take root.

II.5        Innocence of our divine nature (*Avidya*) encourages
            identification with the ever changing, rather than
            with the inner stillness of the heart.

II.6        When undue trust is placed in the individual self
            (*Asmita*), it is confused with the Divine Self.

II.7        Excessive fondness for fleeting pleasures (*Raga*) causes
            longing.

II.8        Excessive avoidance of unpleasant experiences (*Dvesa*)
            causes disdain.

| | |
|---|---|
| II.9 | The elusive awareness of immortality is inherent even for the wise (*Abhinivesah*). |
| II.10 | With keen observation and discretion, these *Kleshas* become translucent. |
| II.11 | If they have manifested into action, the veils must be dissolved through inward practice. |
| II.12 | The womb of karma (*Karmasala*), sheathed by the *Kleshas* (veils), gives birth to experiences now and in the future. |
| II.13 | As long as the veils encase the womb of karma (*Karmasala*), all actions will be affected. |
| II.14 | Karma bears fruits according to the type and quality of the seed planted and the care given to its growth. |
| II.15 | Intuitive Wisdom empowers us to expand beyond the constantly changing natural world (seen) to the abode of the Divine Spirit (seer). |
| II.16 | With this understanding, once-vital difficulties become impotent. |
| II.17 | The source of these difficulties is the inability to recognize the Divine Spirit (seer) as omniscient and therefore separate from the constantly changing natural world (seen). |
| II.18 | When understood as illusory (*Maya*), nature (seen) and her attributes the *gunas* exist to serve the Divine Self (seer) with both enjoyment and liberation. |
| II.19 | These attributes of nature (*gunas*) are both tangible and intangible. |
| II.20 | The Divine Self (seer) observes the world without being affected by it. |
| II.21 | The natural world (seen) exists for the benefit of the Divine Self (seer). |

II.22      With realization of the Divine Self (seer), the illusory
           natural world (seen) becomes transparent, though
           still seemingly very real to those enmeshed in it.

II.23      When the Divine Self (seer) and nature (seen) unite,
           this dynamic and powerful synergy creates the
           illusory world, obscuring the vision of spirit.

II.24      This union is consummated when we forget the Divine
           Self (seer).

II.25      With constant remembrance of the Divine Self, no
           such union is possible.

II.26      Established in the grace of Intuitive Wisdom, we
           experience liberation.

II.27      Liberation is recognized in seven ways: we no longer
           feel the need for knowledge, to stay away from
           anything or anyone, to gather material things, or to
           act, and our constant companions are joy, faith, and
           clarity.

II.28      By embracing *Asthaanga Yoga,* the Eight-Faceted
           Path, Intuitive Wisdom dawns and reveals our inner
           radiance.

II.29      *Asthaanga Yoga,* the Eight-Faceted Path, embraces:

           *Yama:* reflection of our true nature

           *Niyama:* evolution toward harmony

           *Asana:* comfort in being, posture

           *Pranayama:* enhancement and guidance of
           universal *prana* (energy)

           *Pratyahara:* encouraging the senses to draw within

           *Dharana:* gathering and focusing of consciousness
           inward

> *Dhyana*: continuous inward flow of consciousness
>
> *Samadhi*: union with Divine Consciousness

II.30    *Yama* (reflection of our true nature) is experienced through:

> *Ahimsa*: reverence, love, compassion for all
>
> *Satya*: truthfulness, integrity
>
> *Astheya*: generosity, honesty
>
> *Brahmacharya*: balance and moderation of the vital life force
>
> *Aparigraha*: awareness of abundance, fulfillment

II.31    These great truths are universal and inherent to all beings. If they are altered or ignored, the quality of life is greatly compromised.

II.32    *Niyama* (evolution toward harmony) encompasses:

> *Saucha*: simplicity, purity, refinement
>
> *Santosha*: contentment, being at peace with oneself and others
>
> *Tapas*: igniting the purifying flame
>
> *Swadhaya*: sacred study of the Divine through scripture, nature, and introspection
>
> *Iswara Pranidhana*: wholehearted dedication to the Divine

II.33    When presented with disquieting thoughts or feelings, cultivate an opposite, elevated attitude. This is *Pratipaksha Bhavana*.

II.34    The desire to act upon unwholesome thoughts or actions or to cause or condone others toward these thoughts or actions is preventable. This is also *Pratipaksha Bhavana*.

II.35    Embracing reverence and love for all (*Ahimsa*), we
         experience oneness.

II.36    Dedicated to truth and integrity (*Satya*), our thoughts,
         words, and actions gain the power to manifest.

II.37    Abiding in generosity and honesty (*Astheya*), material
         and spiritual prosperity is bestowed.

II.38    Devoted to living a balanced and moderate life
         (*Brahmacharya*), the scope of one's life force
         becomes boundless.

II.39    Acknowledging abundance (*Aparigraha*), we recognize
         the blessings in everything and gain insights into the
         purpose of our worldly existence.

II.40    Through simplicity and continual refinement (*Saucha*),
         the body, thoughts, and emotions become clear
         reflections of the Self within.

II.41    *Saucha* reveals our joyful nature, and the yearning for
         knowing the Self blossoms.

II.42    When at peace and content with oneself and others
         (*Santosha*), supreme joy is celebrated.

II.43    Living life with zeal and sincerity, the purifying flame is
         ignited (*Tapas*), revealing the inner light.

II.44    Sacred study of the Divine through scripture, nature,
         and introspection (*Swadhaya*) guides us to the
         Supreme Self.

II.45    Through wholehearted dedication (*Iswara Pranidhana*),
         we become intoxicated with the Divine.

II.46    The natural comfort and joy of our being is expressed
         when the body becomes steady (*Asana*).

II.47    As the body yields all efforts and holdings, the infinite
         within is revealed.

II.48     Thereafter we are freed from the fluctuations of the
          *gunas*.

II.49     The universal life force (*prana*) is enhanced and guided
          through the harmonious rhythm of the breath
          (*Pranayama*).

II.50     The movement of the life force is influenced by
          inhalation, exhalation, and sustained breath.

II.51     A balanced, rhythmic pattern steadies the mind and
          emotions, causing the breath to become motionless.

II.52     As a result, the veils over the inner light are lifted.

II.53     The vista of higher consciousness is revealed.

II.54     Encouraging the senses to draw inward is *Pratyahara*.

II.55     Glimpsing the inner light, the senses contentedly dwell
          within.

III.1     Gathering consciousness and focusing it within is
          *Dharana* (contemplation).

III.2     The continuous inward flow of consciousness is
          *Dhyana* (meditation).

III.3     When individual consciousness unites with the Divine
          Consciousness, the illusion of separateness dissolves;
          this is *Samadhi*.

III.4     When *Dharana* (contemplation), *Dhyana* (meditation),
          and *Samadhi* (union with Divine Consciousness)
          seamlessly merge into one another, this is *Samyama*
          (fusion).

III.5     Through *Samyama*, individual and Divine
          Consciousness gracefully reunite.

III.6     The insights and wisdom gained through *Samyama*
          enhance all aspects of life.

III.7          The three facets that comprise *Samyama* (*Dharana*, *Dhyana*, and *Samadhi*) are more subtle than the preceding five.

III.8          Even these three facets that make up *Samyama* appear external when the seedless *Samadhi* (*Nirbija*) is experienced.

III.9          By observing the silent moments that occur between the rising thoughts and feelings without controlling them, consciousness is transformed and expanded (*Nirodha Parinama*).

III.10         As the transformation of consciousness (*Nirodha Parinama*) becomes steady, profound tranquility is experienced.

III.11         Then the fluctuations of consciousness are pacified, and *Samadhi* (*Samadhi Parinama*) becomes a familiar state of being.

III.12         From this all thoughts and feelings, without divergence, flow into captivated awareness (*Ekagrata Parinama*).

III.13         Through the three phases of *Samyama,* the natural elements are transformed, as are the thoughts, feelings, and senses, securing and expanding the state of higher consciousness.

III.14         An object possessing the external attributes of nature (*gunas*) remains subject to constant change, revealing the past, present, or yet to be manifested.

III.15         The progression of these attributes of nature is the cause of constant changes in our ongoing evolution.

III.16         From *Samyama* on the advancing of time comes knowledge of past and future.

III.17         A word, its meaning, and the idea behind it are often confused because of their superimposition upon one another. By *Samyama* on the word or sound, knowledge of its meaning is revealed.

III.18    Through *Samyama* on past impressions, knowledge of previous births is granted.

III.19    Through purity of consciousness, one gains the ability to understand the nature of their own mind and also those of others.

III.20    Understanding the nature of another's thoughts and feelings gives us insight into the contents and motives beyond them.

III.21    By *Samyama* on the subtle body, one gains the power to intercept the light emanating from their body before it reaches the eyes of the observer; therefore the yogi's body becomes invisible.

III.22    In the same way as described above, one is able to intercept the outward manifestation of the senses of smell, taste, hearing, and touch, so they become undetectable to others.

III.23    By *Samyama* on two aspects of karma (instantaneous and delayed), knowledge of the fruits of our actions will be revealed, along with time of death.

III.24    By *Samyama* on kindness and other virtuous qualities, one develops the power to transmit those qualities to others.

III.25    By *Samyama* on strength, we experience the level of vigor of elephants.

III.26    By *Samyama* on the inner light in the heart, one is granted powers of deep perception.

III.27    By *Samyama* on the sun, knowledge of the inner and outer worlds is revealed.

III.28    By *Samyama* on the moon, we gain knowledge of the stars and galaxies as well as the subtle aspects of our being.

III.29    By *Samyama* on the polestar (*Dhruva Nakshatra*) comes
          knowledge of the celestial movements and their
          effects on the events of this world.

III.30    By *Samyama* on the navel, one acquires knowledge of
          how the human body functions and its constitution.

III.31    By *Samyama* at the base of the throat, the cessation of
          hunger and thirst is achieved.

III.32    By *Samyama* at the base of the throat, steadiness in
          meditation for both body and mind is accomplished.

III.33    By *Samyama* on the light radiating from the center of
          the head, visions of celestial and enlightened beings
          are bestowed.

III.34    Or all these powers and the knowledge within them
          may be imparted to those who become spontaneously
          enlightened through a life of purity.

III.35    By *Samyama* on the spiritual heart (*Hridaya*), the intent
          and contents of the *chitta* are revealed.

III.36    Through *Samyama* we are able to distinguish between
          the *chitta* and the True Self.

III.37    From this knowledge arise all our supernatural senses,
          which correspond to the external senses of sight,
          hearing, touch, taste, and smell.

III.38    While considered to be great accomplishments, these
          occult senses can be obstacles to reaching *Samadhi*
          and higher consciousness.

III.39    Through loosening the bonds of karma, one can leave
          their body at will or even enter another's body.

III.40    By *Samyama* on the element of air, levitation over all
          naturally occurring objects, including water and land,
          becomes possible. It also grants the ability to die at
          will.

III.41      By *Samyama* on the solar plexus, the element of fire, housed there, causes the *samana vayu* (the equalizing vital air) to produce a radiant aura that surrounds the body.

III.42      By *Samyama* on the relationship between space and sound, one acquires the power of hearing distant and divine sounds; supernormal hearing (clairaudience) becomes possible.

III.43      By *Samyama* on the relationship between the body and ether, weightlessness and levitation are attained and traveling through space becomes possible.

III.44      By *Samyama* on consciousness (*Mahavideha*), the *chitta* acts independently from the physical body, causing the veil over the inner light of the Self to become transparent.

III.45      By *Samyama* on the basic and subtle characteristics of the natural elements and the *gunas* that comprise them, their purpose is revealed, and one gains mastery over them.

III.46      By gaining mastery over the natural elements, one is no longer subjected to their play or the obstacles they impose on the physical body, allowing the eight supernatural powers to manifest.

III.47      Achieving this mastery, the physical body reveals beauty and grace, combined with solidity and strength.

III.48      By *Samyama* on the transformation that the senses undergo when they contact objects, and the experience they provide for the individual, mastery over the senses is gained.

III.49      Thus the body gains the power to move as rapidly as thought, and the sense organs engage outside the confines of the body, enabling mastery over the aspects of nature (*Prakriti*).

III.50    By recognizing the distinction between the *chitta* and
          the True Self, one gains knowledge of everything that
          exists and all that manifests within nature (*Prakriti*).

III.51    After acquiring all these *siddhis,* if we renounce them,
          embracing only the Divine Self, liberation follows.

III.52    Dwelling in a state of equanimity, the yogi neither
          accepts nor rejects admiration from others, even
          celestial beings; thus their heart stays pure and
          embraces only the Divine.

III.53    By *Samyama* on the smallest moment, as well as the
          succession of moments of time, the knowledge of
          supreme liberation is attained.

III.54    With this exalted knowledge, the yogi is able to clearly
          distinguish even the most minute differences
          between two similar objects.

III.55    This intuitive knowledge, which has the ability to
          comprehend all objects under various conditions
          simultaneously, leads us to freedom.

III.56    Liberation is attained when the spiritual heart
          (*Hridaya*) attains purity equal to that of the True
          Self.

IV.1      *Siddhis* (powers) manifest through spiritual practices
          performed in previous births or through the use of
          herbs, mantra repetition, asceticism, or immersion in
          *Samadhi*.

IV.2      Due to the transforming power of spiritual practices,
          nature's energy flows with such abundance that it
          aids the spiritual seeker's evolution toward gaining a
          higher birth.

IV.3      While the practices do not directly affect
          transformation, they act to prevent obstacles from
          blocking the flow of nature's energy, needed for
          liberation.

IV.4    Identification with the individual self (*Asmita*) creates the *chitta* and its myriad thoughts and emotions.

IV.5    Under certain conditions consciousness branches into many different types of thoughts, feelings, or actions. This is rooted in a mistaken sense of individuality rather than the true source of oneness.

IV.6    Through deep meditation the *chitta* becomes impotent and one becomes free from karma.

IV.7    The actions (karmas) of the yogi, transformed through *Dhyana*, meditation, are neutralized and are therefore neither good nor bad, while the actions of others are still categorized as either good, bad, or mixed.

IV.8    When those three types of actions (karmas) have favorable conditions, they create impressions that have the ability to manifest at any moment in time.

IV.9    Because memory holds on to past impressions, the chain of cause and effect (karma) remains intact from one life to the next, as if there were no separation between births.

IV.10   These past impressions are created without beginning or end, fueling the perpetual cycle of birth and death and the desire for immortality.

IV.11   Impressions and desires that manifest because of the veils covering the inner light (*Kleshas*) are bound together by cause and effect. Resolving back into seed form, they cease to function.

IV.12   Both past and future simultaneously exist in all objects, while exhibiting different characteristics due to the movements of nature (*gunas*).

IV.13   Past, present, and future, whether manifested or subtle, are caused by fluctuation of the *gunas*.

IV.14     When they are unbalanced, the play of the *gunas* cause
          modifications in an object, but if they are in balance,
          the unique essence and expression of the object does
          not change.

IV.15     Due to differences in understanding and the various
          ways one perceives objects and actions, each person
          may view the same object differently, according to
          their own perception.

IV.16     Therefore, the object is not dependent on a single
          perception. Otherwise, the object would be said to be
          nonexistent if that one individual is not perceiving it.

IV.17     The essence of an object is known or unknown
          according to the conditioning or expectation of the
          individual consciousness perceiving it.

IV.18     The Seer, being omniscient, observes the changes and
          transformations taking place within the thoughts and
          emotions.

IV.19     Knowledge and perception can be experienced only by
          the Seer, as the *chitta* is not self-luminous.

IV.20     Without the inner light, the *chitta* is unable to perceive
          both subject and object simultaneously.

IV.21     The various thoughts and feelings contained in the
          *chitta* are reflections of a single consciousness that is
          all-knowing and unchangeable.

IV.22     When pure consciousness illuminates the *chitta*, it
          simulates the reflections and characteristics of
          that consciousness, causing the *chitta* to appear
          conscious.

IV.23     The *chitta,* in order to distinguish an object of
          perception, must assume knowledge from the one
          consciousness.

IV.24      Though having countless desires, the *chitta* seeks not
           only to satisfy the senses but also to further the
           emancipation of the soul.

IV.25      By increased discrimination, the *chitta* ceases to
           identify itself as the Divine Consciousness.

IV.26      Then the *chitta*, enticed toward discrimination, propels
           itself into liberation.

IV.27      If discrimination becomes lax, distractions due to past
           impressions may arise.

IV.28      These distractions from enlightenment can be
           redirected through inward practices in the same
           manner as we dissolve the veils over the inner light,
           the *Kleshas*.

IV.29      Through the grace of Intuitive Wisdom, one remains
           totally disinterested even in the possession of all the
           psychic powers and ascends to the Cloud of Virtue
           (*Dharmamegha Samadhi*).

IV.30      Reaching the exalted state of *Dharmamegha Samadhi*
           (the Cloud of Virtue), all sufferings and karmas
           cease.

IV.31      Upon realization of this infinite knowledge, the entire
           universe, with all its sense objects, loses its powers of
           attraction.

IV.32      The *gunas*, having fulfilled their purpose, become
           impotent.

IV.33      In the final stages of liberation, the fluctuation of the
           *gunas* ceases to function, causing time to become
           irrelevant.

IV.34      *Kaivalya*, liberation, manifests as the impotent *gunas*
           reabsorb themselves into *Prakriti* (nature), revealing
           the exalted consciousness shining forth as Divine
           Light.

# ACKNOWLEDGMENTS

## With Gratitude

It was the women, so many of them over the years, who encouraged and, yes, at times cajoled me to take on this momentous project. My heart wanted to keep my way of seeing the teachings nestled within it. "You have to write this book for us," they told me. Now that it is birthed, my gratitude is wrapped in their eagerness for the sutras representing them, in "their language."

The numerous nameless faces come back to me as I begin to pour out my gratitude, the magnitude of which cannot begin to be expressed. My hope is that in naming a few I will also recognize the others.

I begin with my mother, whose faith in me was unwavering; in her eyes and heart, I could do *anything*. Although being a woman in her lifetime may have hindered *her* way of life, she made sure the prejudices did not funnel my life into small thinking. My father by his example showed me that following your own heart was not always popular but was the only way to live.

With gratitude I honor all my teachers, formal and informal, who brought the scriptures, especially the Yoga Sutras, to life for me. Sri Swami Satchidanandaji, whose clear and simple yet profound way of telling them enabled me to absorb them immediately into a new way of living. Mataji Indra Devi and other teachers, who continued to inspire me through either their example or their writings.

To all the students I taught, who experienced the heart of the Yoga

Sutras and reflected their experiences back to me. Encouraging me, they chanted, *"You* are the one to write this book!"

This project was infused with much masculine support, from the male students, who wanted another, more heartfelt voice to the sutras, to my soul mate, Bhaskar Deva, who allowed himself to be educated as to the prejudices and inhibition of the feminine power, saying, "That many women were persecuted! I had no idea. This is important; you must add this to the book!" His unwavering love keeps me in my heart.

David Frawley (Pandit Vamadeva Shastri), a great modern-day pundit, encouraged me to "tell the sutras from the heart," affirming to me that *chitta* means heart, not mind.

The mystical gratitude is less easy to express. While at the computer, surrounded by all the aspects of the feminine Divine I could find, I was constantly playing the Saraswati (goddess of wisdom and knowledge) mantra. The goddess Saraswati (and Vak, goddess of speech) has been my constant companion and spirit writer in this awesome outpouring of love. I know that without divine grace, this book would not have been possible.

Read the sutras; meditate on them; experience their true meaning. If you do this with your heart, you will know newfound enrichment in your Yoga practice, and in everything you do.

May we live in love and joy realizing our own divine nature. Om Shanti, Shanti, Shanti.

# INDEX

feelings (emotions), 30, 68, 104,
    107, 128, 158, 159, 163, 166,
    190, 204
  *Bhakti* devotion and, 65
  controlling, 18–19
  devoted practice and, 48
  *gunas* and, 58–62
  habits of, 31–32
  *Hatha Yoga* and, 236, 239, 241,
    243, 245, 247–248
  identifying with, 27–28
  imagination and, 30, 38–39
  insight and, 300
  kindness and, 87
  language and, 224
  misunderstanding and, 37–38
  moon and, 60–61
  *Nirodha Parinama* and, 288
  perception, 384–385, 386–389
  *Pratipaksha Bhavana* and, 174,
    181–184
  refinement of, 215, 216–219
  *Samyama* and, 289, 292, 294,
    295, 297–298
  *Tapas* and, 121
  thoughts and, xxxii–xxxiv
  as wind, 21–22
"fight or flight" syndrome, 197–198
Fleming, Alexander, 228
forgiveness, 37–38, 92
freedom. *See* liberation

Galileo Galilei, 36, 229
Gandhi, Mahatma, 90, 189–190,
    202, 207
Gayatri Mantra, 115–123
generosity. *See Astheya*
Golden Age (*Sat Yuga*), xxvii–xxix,
    152, 178, 179, 188, 190, 236
gossip, 197–198
grace, 32, 68, 81, 101, 103, 105
gratitude. *See Aparigraha*
*Grihastha*, 209

guilt, 56
*gunas*, 14–16, 45, 57–62, 78, 106,
    145–146, 234, 236, 252–253
  change and, 299, 301
  as hindrances, 361, 378–387
  Intuitive Wisdom and, 156,
    158–160, 162, 163
  mastery, 336, 343–347, 396
  tangible and intangible, 157,
    162–163
gurus and teachers, 71–75, 91,
    227–228, 294, 308, 330

habits. *See Samskaras*
harming, 91–92, 185–186, 190,
    191, 192
*Hatha Yoga*, 19–20, 65, 234–258
  asanas in, 19, 43, 50, 315–316
heart(s). *See also* love
  as crystal, 96, 98–100
  devoted practice and, 45,
    48–50, 81–82, 84, 94–95, 224,
    272–274
  inner light, 300, 317
  language of the heart, xxii–xxvii
  learning by heart, xxxi–xxxiv
  lightness of, 221
  open, xxxvi, 12–13, 15, 65–66,
    70–71, 81–82, 87, 88, 93, 148,
    181–182, 190–191, 200–201,
    202, 217–218, 306, 312–313
  *Samyama* and, o270
  spiritual (*Hridaya*), 300, 317, 319,
    329–332, 354, 358–359
  uniting of consciousness in, 17,
    18–24
  wisdom from, 159
  of women, 67–69
herbs, 363, 365, 366
Hillel, Rabbi, 228
honesty, 187, 199–202
*Hridaya*, 300, 317, 319, 329–332,
    354, 358–359

# ABOUT THE AUTHOR

© Kelly Love Ross

NISCHALA JOY DEVI is a master teacher and healer. For many years she has been highly respected as an international advocate for her innovative way of expressing Yoga and its subtle uses for spiritual growth and complete healing.

She was a monastic student of the world-renowned Yogiraj Sri Swami Satchidananda and spent more than twenty-five years receiving his direct guidance and teachings. During her time in the monastery, she began to blend Western medicine with Yoga and meditation. She then offered her expertise in developing the Yoga portion of the Dean Ornish Program for Reversing Heart Disease, where she subsequently served as director of Stress Management. She also cofounded the award-winning Commonweal Cancer Help Program.

Nischala Devi produced the "Abundant Well-Being Series" CDs to allow these simple yet profound Yoga and stress-relieving techniques to reach more people. Her book *The Healing Path of Yoga* also expresses these teachings.

With her knowledge of Yoga and her experience in assisting those with life-threatening diseases, she created *Yoga of the Heart,* a training and certification program for Yoga teachers and health professionals designed to adapt Yoga practices to the special needs of that population.

Passionate about the field of Yoga Therapy, she was one of the founders of the International Association of Yoga Therapists, and serves on the advisory board. With this vision she created a series of online classes to allow aspiring yogis and therapists to further their knowledge in different aspects of healing.

Understanding the need for more love and compassion in today's world, *The Namaste Effect* explores a heart-centered way of living through the mystical chakras.

Highlighting her passion for the more subtle teachings of Yoga, she wrote *Meditation in the Yoga Tradition* to aid those looking to delve deeper into their spiritual nature.

She is dedicated to bringing the Feminine back into spirituality and the scriptures in her book *The Secret Power of Yoga,* a woman's guide to the heart and spirit of the Yoga Sutras and *The Secret Power of Yoga* audiobook (Nautilus Book Award winner).

For information on programs, training, and retreats, please visit her website, www.abundantwellbeing.com.

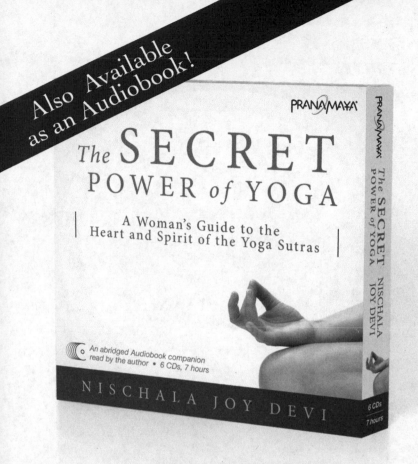